The Starvation Treatment of Diabetes

By Lewis Webb Hill and Rena S. Eckman

INTRODUCTION.

Although Dr. Allen's modifications of the classical treatment of saccharine diabetes have been in use only for about two years in the hands of their author, and for a much shorter time in those of other physicians, it seems to me already clearly proven that Dr. Allen has notably advanced our ability to combat the disease.

One of the difficulties which is likely to prevent the wide adoption of his treatment is the detailed knowledge of food composition and calorie value which it requires. Dr. Hill's and Miss Eckman's little book should afford substantial aid to all who have not had opportunity of working out in detail the progressive series of diets which should be used after the starvation period. These diets, worked out by Miss Eckman, head of the diet kitchen at the Massachusetts General Hospital, have seemed to me to work admirably with the patients who have taken them, both in hospital and private practice. The use of thrice boiled vegetables, as recommended by Dr. Allen, seems to be a substantial step in advance, giving, as it does, a considerable bulk of food without any considerable carbohydrate portion, and with the semblance of some of the forbidden vegetables.

It is, of course, too early to say how far reaching and how permanent the effects of such a diet will be in the severe and in the milder cases of diabetes. All we can say is that thus far it appears to work admirably well. To all who wish to give their patients the benefit of this treatment I can heartily recommend this book.

Richard C. Cabot.

PREFACE TO FIRST EDITION.

The purpose of this little book is to furnish to the general practitioner in compact form the details of the latest and most successful treatment of diabetes mellitus.

The "starvation treatment" of diabetes, as advanced by Dr. Frederick M. Allen of the Rockefeller Institute Hospital, is undoubtedly a most valuable treatment. At the Massachusetts General Hospital it has been used for several months with great success, and it is thought worth while to publish some of the diets, and details of treatment that have been used there, as a very careful control of the proteid and carbohydrate intake is of the utmost importance if the treatment is to be successful. In carrying out the Allen treatment the physician must think in grams of carbohydrate and proteid--it is not enough simply to cut down the supply of starchy foods; he must know approximately how much carbohydrate and proteid his patient is getting each day. It is not easy for a busy practitioner to figure out these dietary values, and for this reason the calculated series of diets given here may be of service. The various tests for sugar, acetone, etc., can, of course, be found in any good text-book of chemistry, but it is thought worth while to include them here for the sake of completeness and ready reference. The food table covers most of the ordinary foods.

We wish to thank Dr. Roger I. Lee and Dr. William H. Smith, visiting physicians, for many helpful suggestions.

PREFACE TO SECOND EDITION.

The Authors beg to thank the Profession for the cordial reception given the first edition of this book. The present edition has been revised and enlarged, with the addition of considerable new material which we hope will be of use.

January, 1916.

DETAILS OF TREATMENT

DETAILS OF TREATMENT.

For forty-eight hours after admission to the hospital the patient is kept on ordinary diet, to determine the severity of his diabetes. Then he is starved, and no food allowed save whiskey and black coffee. The whiskey is given in the coffee: 1 ounce of whiskey every two hours, from 7 A.M. until 7 P.M. This furnishes roughly about 800 calories. The whiskey is not an essential part of the treatment; it merely furnishes a few calories and keeps the patient more comfortable while he is being starved. If it is not desired to give whiskey, bouillon or any clear soup may be given instead. The water intake need not be restricted. Soda bicarbonate may be given, two drachms every three hours, if there is much evidence of acidosis, as indicated by strong acetone and diacetic acid reactions in the urine, or a strong acetone odor to the breath. In most cases, however, this is not at all necessary, and there is no danger of producing coma by the starvation. This is indeed the most important point that Dr. Allen has brought out in his treatment. At first it was thought best to keep patients in bed during the fast, but it is undoubtedly true that most patients do better and become sugar-free more quickly if they are up and around, taking a moderate amount of exercise for at least a part of the day. Starvation is continued until the urine shows no sugar. (The daily weight and daily urine examinations are, of course, recorded.) The disappearance of the sugar is rapid: if there has been 5 or 6 per cent., after the first starvation day it goes down to perhaps 2 per cent., and the next day the patient may be entirely sugar-free or perhaps have .2 or .3 per cent. of sugar. Occasionally it may take longer; the longest we have starved any patient is four days, but we know of obstinate cases that have been starved for as long as ten or eleven days without bad results. The patients tolerate starvation remarkably well; in no cases have we seen any ill effects from it. There may be a slight loss of weight, perhaps three or four pounds, but this is of no moment, and indeed, Allen says that a moderate loss of weight in most diabetics is to be desired. A moderately obese patient, weighing say 180 pounds, may continue to excrete a small amount of sugar for a considerable period if he holds this weight, even if he is taking very little carbohydrate; whereas, if his weight can be reduced to 170 or 160, he can be kept sugar-free, with ease, on the same diet. This is very important: reduce the weight of a fat diabetic, and keep it reduced.

We have not found that the acetone and diacetic acid output behaves in any constant manner during starvation; in some cases we have seen the acetone bodies disappear, in others we have seen them appear when they were not present before.

Their appearance is not necessarily a cause for alarm. The estimation of the ammonia in the urine is of some value in determining the amount of acidosis present, and this can readily be done by the simple chemical method given below. If the 24-hourly ammonia output reaches over 3 or 4 grams, it means that there is a good deal of acidosis--anything below this is not remarkable. More exact methods of determining the amount of acidosis are the determination of the ratio between the total urinary nitrogen and the ammonia, the quantitation of the acetone, diacetic acid and oxy-butyric acid excreted, and the carbon dioxide tension of the alveolar air. These are rather complicated for average clinical use, however.

When the patient is sugar-free he is put upon a diet of so-called "5% vegetables," i.e. vegetables containing approximately 5% carbohydrate. It is best to boil these vegetables three times, with changes of water. In this way their carbohydrate content is reduced, probably about one-half. A moderate amount of fat, in the form of butter, can be given with this vegetable diet if desired. The amount of carbohydrate in these green vegetables is not at all inconsiderable, and if the patient eats as much as he desires, it is possible for him to have an intake of 25 or 30 grams, which is altogether too much; the first day after starvation the carbohydrate intake should not be over 15 grams. Tables No. 1 and No. 2 represent these vegetable diets. The patient is usually kept on diet 1 or 2 for one day, or if the case is a particularly severe one, for two days. The day after the vegetable day, the protein and fat are raised, the carbohydrate being left at the same figure (diets 2, 3 and 4). No absolute rule can be laid down for the length of time for a patient to remain on one diet, but in general we do not give the very low diets such as 2, 3 and 4, for more than a day or two at a time. The diet should be raised very gradually, and it is not well to raise the protein and carbohydrate at the same time, for it is important to know which of the two is causing the more trouble. The protein intake may perhaps be raised more rapidly than the carbohydrate, but an excess of protein is very important in causing glycosuria, and for this reason the protein intake must be watched as carefully as the carbohydrate. With adults, it is advisable to give about 1 gram of protein per kilogram of body weight, if possible; with children 1.5 to 2 grams. It will be noticed that the diets which follow contain rather small amounts of fat, a good deal less than is usually given to diabetics. There are two reasons for this: In the first place, we do not want our diabetics, our adults, at any rate, to gain weight; and in the second place acidosis is much easier to get rid of if the fat intake is kept low. If the fat values given in the diets are found too low for any individual case, fat can very easily be added in the form of butter, cream or bacon. Most adults do well on about 30 calories per kilogram of body weight; children of four years need 75 calories per kilogram, children of eight years need 60, and children of twelve years need 50.

If sugar appears in the urine during the process of raising the diet, we drop back to a lower diet, and if this is unavailing, start another starvation day, and raise the diet more slowly. But it will be found, if the diet is raised very slowly, sugar will not appear. It is not well to push the average case; if the patient is taking a fair diet, say protein 50, carbohydrate 50 and fat 150, and is doing well, without any glycosuria, it is not desirable to raise the diet any further. The caloric intake may seem rather low in some of these diets, but it is surprising to see how well most patients do on 1500 or 2000 calories.

It will be seen that the treatment can be divided into three stages:

(1) The stage of starvation, when the patient is becoming sugar-free.

(2) The stage of gradually working up the diet to the limit of tolerance.

During the first two stages a daily weight record should be kept, and the urine should be examined every day. The patient should, of course, be under the immediate supervision of the physician during these two stages. It is always well to discharge a patient on a diet somewhat under his tolerance, if possible.

(3) The stationary stage, when the diet is kept at a constant level. The patient is at home and going about his business. Most patients may be taught to test their own urine, and they should do this every other day. If there is sugar in the urine, the patient should go back to a lower diet, and if he cannot be made sugar-free this way, he should be starved again. A semi-starvation day of 150 grams of vegetables, once a week, whether or no the urine contains sugar, is of value for the purpose of keeping well within the margin of safety and of reminding the patient that he is on a strict diet.

It is very important for a diabetic to take a considerable amount of exercise: he can utilize his carbohydrate better, if he does.

If this treatment is to be successful, it is absolutely necessary for the patient to adhere very strictly to the diets, and to measure out everything very carefully; the meat especially should be weighed.

It will be noticed that in some cases the calories in the diets do not tally exactly with the protein, fat and carbohydrate values. The reason for this is that for the sake of convenience the calories have been given in round numbers--5 or ten calories one way or the other makes no difference.

The essential points brought out by Allen's treatment are as follows:

(1) It is not dangerous to starve a diabetic, and two or three days of starvation almost always make a patient sugar-free, thus saving a good deal of time, as contrasted with the old treatment of gradually cutting down the carbohydrate.

(2) It is not desirable for all diabetics to hold their weight. Some cases may do much better if their weight is reduced ten, fifteen, or even twenty pounds.

(3) After starvation, the diet must be raised very slowly, to prevent recurrence of glycosuria.

(4) An excess of protein must be regarded as producing glycosuria and an excess of fat ketonuria, and the protein and fat intake must be restricted a good deal more than has usually been the custom in treating diabetes.

Case Reports.

It is thought worth while, for the sake of illustration, to include a few case reports. The adults were treated at the Massachusetts General Hospital, the children at the Children's Hospital.

Two charts are kept for each case: one a food chart, with the amounts of the different articles of food taken each day, and the protein, carbohydrate, fat and caloric value figured out for each foodstuff; the second (see below) a more general chart, which shows graphically the progress of the case.

The first three are cases which were treated first with the old method of gradually reducing the carbohydrate intake and could never be made sugar-free, running from 0.1% to 0.2% of sugar. On the new treatment they responded promptly and were discharged sugar-free.

* * * * *

Case 1. A woman of 64, diabetic for two years. She was sent in from the out-patient department, where she had been receiving a diet of 50 grams of carbohydrate and 50 grams of protein. On this diet she was putting out 8 grams of sugar a day with moderately strong acetone and diacetic acid reactions in her urine. When the carbohydrate was cut in the ward to 30 grams, she put out 3 grams of sugar a day. She complained of severe pruritus vulvae. After sixteen days of this treatment she continued to put out from 0.1% to 0.2% of sugar a day. Allen's treatment was then started, and after one day of starvation she was sugar-free and remained so for four days on a diet of carbohydrate, 20 grams; protein, 30 grams; fat, 150 grams. The itching had gone. Then the protein was raised to 80 grams, with the carbohydrate at 20 grams, and she immediately showed 1.5% of sugar. This is very important; the protein should not be raised too quickly. This we did not realize in our earlier cases.

A second starvation day, followed by two vegetable days, and a more careful raising of the diet--as follows--kept her sugar-free, and she was discharged so. Her diets were:

Dec. 12. Carbohydrate, 20 grams. Protein, 30 grams. Fat, 150 grams--1500 calories. No glycosuria.

Dec. 15. Carbohydrate, 30 grams. Protein, 30 grams. Fat, 200 grams--2000 calories. No glycosuria.

Dec. 20. Carbohydrate, 30 grams. Protein, 40 grams. Fat, 180 grams--2000 calories. No glycosuria.

Dec. 26. Carbohydrate, 40 grams. Protein, 40 grams. Fat, 180 grams 2000 calories. No glycosuria.

Dec. 30. Carbohydrates, 50 grams. Protein, 50 grams. Fat, 180 grams--2000 calories. No glycosuria. Weight on entrance, 119 pounds. Weight at discharge, 116 pounds.

* * * * *

Case 2. A Jew of 49, at entrance had 175 grams of sugar (5.5%), acetone slight, diacetic acid absent. Treated for three weeks with the old method, he got down to a diet containing carbohydrate, 15 grams; protein, 50 grams,-- but still put out from 3 to 8 grams of sugar a day. By the old method we could not do away with the last traces of sugar.

The Allen treatment was started with two starvation days. On the second he was sugar-free--but showed 2.6 grams of sugar the following day on 12 grams of carbohydrate and 40 grams of protein. (This was one of the earlier cases when the diet was raised too quickly after starvation.) After one more starvation day and two vegetable days he stayed sugar-free while the diet was raised slowly to 30 grams of carbohydrate and 45 grams of protein, calories about 2000. Discharged sugar-free on this diet.

Weight at entrance, 109 pounds. Weight at discharge, 110 pounds.

* * * * *

Case 3. A man of 35, a severe diabetic, entered Dec. 28, 1914. He had been in the hospital the previous July for a month and could never be made sugar-free with the old method of treatment. At entrance he was putting out 2.5% of sugar (135 grams) per day with strongly positive acetone and diacetic acid tests. Two starvation days made him sugar-free, but we made the mistake of not using twice boiled vegetables for his vegetable day after starvation. So on this day he got about 30 grams of carbohydrates, and for a few days he showed from 0.2% to 1% of sugar. Another starvation day was given him and he became sugar-free. This time his vegetables were closely restricted and he was given only enough twice-boiled vegetables to provide about 15 grams of carbohydrates. After this the diet was raised very slowly. He remained sugar-free for three weeks and was discharged so on,

Carbohydrate, 20 grams. Protein, 40 grams. Fat, 200 grams. At no time did he receive more than 2200 calories. Weight at entrance, 139 pounds. Weight at discharge, 138 pounds.

* * * * *

These three cases were the first ones we tried, and in each one of them we made the mistake of raising the diet too quickly--either allowing too many vegetables on the vegetable day, or raising the protein too quickly afterwards. With the later cases, after we had more experience, there was no more trouble.

* * * * *

Case 4. A Greek (male) of 48, diabetic for two months, entered Jan. 14, 1915, with 3.8% (65 grams) of sugar and moderate acetone reaction. There was no diacetic reaction present at entrance. After one starvation day he became sugar-free, but was kept on starvation one day longer and then started on vegetables in the usual way. After the third day a moderate amount of diacetic acid appeared in the urine and continued. The ammonia rose from 0.7 grams per day to 2.6 grams per day, and then varied from 0.3 to 1.5 grams per day. No symptoms of acidosis.

Jan. 18. Carbohydrate, 15 grams. Protein, 25 grams. Fat, 150 grams--1360 calories. No glycosuria.

Jan. 20. Carbohydrate, 15 grams. Protein, 25 grams. Fat, 200 grams--1571 calories. No glycosuria.

Jan. 24. Carbohydrate, 25 grams. Protein, 35 grams. Fat, 200 grams--1760 calories. No glycosuria.

Jan. 26. Carbohydrate, 35 grams. Protein, 40 grams. Fat, 200 grams--1838 calories. No glycosuria.

Jan. 29. Carbohydrate, 45 grams. Protein, 50 grams. Fat, 200 grams--2194 calories. No glycosuria.

Jan. 31. Carbohydrate, 50 grams. Protein, 60 grams. Fat, 200 grams--2347 calories. No glycosuria. Discharged Feb. 1 sugar-free on this diet. Weight at entrance, 160 pounds. Weight at discharge, 156 pounds. This was not a severe case and responded very easily to treatment.

* * * * *

Case 5. A female of 59, a diabetic of two years' standing, excreted 2.6% of sugar on Jan. 16, 1915, with no acetone or diacetic acid reactions in the urine. Severe pruritus vulvae. Starved two days; sugar-free on the second starvation day, with disappearance of the pruritus.

Jan. 21. Carbohydrate, 15 grams. Protein, 25 grams. Fat, 150 grams--1595 calories. No glycosuria. From this time the diet was slowly raised until on

Jan. 30 she was getting Carbohydrate, 35 grams. Protein, 45 grams. Fat, 200 grams--2156 calories. She was sugar-free on this and was discharged to the out-patient department after a two weeks' stay in the wards. Weight at entrance, 135 pounds. Weight at discharge, 133 pounds.

* * * * *

Case 6. A man of 52, entered Jan. 10, 1915, with 1% of sugar. He entered for arteriosclerosis and hypertension, and the sugar was found in the routine examination of the urine. He was kept on house diet for a few days and his sugar rose to 3.5%. No acetone or diacetic acid. After two days of starvation he became sugar-free and continued so as the diet was slowly raised. He was kept sugar-free in the ward eighteen days and was sugar-free on Feb. 6 with a diet of

Carbohydrate, 60 grams. Protein, 60 grams. Fat, 200 grams--2280 calories.

On Feb. 7 the protein was raised to 80 grams and 0.2% of sugar appeared in the urine. The protein was then reduced to 60 grams and he remained sugar-free on this diet and was discharged so.

In this case, after starvation, a moderate amount of acetone appeared and continued. No symptoms of acidosis. The ammonia ran from 0.3 to 1.0 grams per day.

Weight at entrance, 160 pounds. Weight after three weeks' treatment, 156. Maximum caloric intake, 2525.

* * * * *

Case 7. A young man of 25, diabetic for eight months, entered Jan. 20, 1915, with 6.6% (112 grams) of sugar and strongly positive tests for acetone and diacetic acid. After a period of two starvation days he was sugar-free and actually gained three pounds in the process of starvation (probably due to water retention).

His diet was then raised as follows:--

Jan. 24. Carbohydrate, 15 grams. Protein, 25 grams. Fat, 150 grams. No glycosuria.

Jan. 26. Carbohydrate, 20 grams. Protein, 35 grams. Fat, 175 grams. No glycosuria.

Jan. 29. Carbohydrate, 20 grams. Protein, 45 grams. Fat, 200 grams. No glycosuria.

Jan. 31. Carbohydrate, 30 grams. Protein, 45 grams. Fat, 200 grams. No glycosuria.

At entrance his ammonia was 1.7 grams per day; after the starvation days it ran from 0.9 grams to 0.3 grams per day. The acetone was a little stronger than at entrance; the diacetic absent except on three days.

On Feb. 5 he was still sugar-free having been so since his starvation days two weeks previously, and weighed 127 pounds, a gain of seven pounds since entrance. At no time did he receive over 2150 calories.

This was a very satisfactory case; no doubt the carbohydrate could have been raised to 50 or 60 grams, but he was doing so well that we felt It unwise to go any further.

* * * * *

Diabetes in children is likely to be a good deal more severe than it is in adults. Still, in the few cases that have been treated with the starvation treatment at the Children's Hospital, the results have been very satisfactory, as far as rendering the patient sugar-free is concerned. Most diabetic children, however, are thin and frail, and they have no extra weight to lose, so it does not seem so desirable to bring about any very great loss of weight, which is quite an essential part of the treatment for most adults. The few children that have been treated have borne starvation remarkably well. It is too early, and we have seen too few children treated by this method, to say what influence it may have on the course of the disease, but it can certainly be said that it is very efficacious in rendering them sugar-free.

* * * * *

Case 8. M. M., female, 12 years, entered the Children's Hospital April 1, 1915. She had probably had diabetes for about 6 months, and had been on a general diet at home. (See charts on pp. 31-36.)

On the ordinary diet of the ward she showed 8.7% sugar, no acetone or diacetic acid. Weight, 52-1/4 pounds,--a very thin, frail girl. She was starved two days, taking about 1-1/2 oz. of whiskey in black coffee each day.

The first day of starvation the sugar dropped to 2.3%, and a slight trace of acetone appeared in the urine. The second day of starvation she was sugar-free, with a moderate acetone reaction. No soda bicarbonate was given. She lost 2 pounds during starvation. After she became sugar-free, her diets were as follows:

April 5. Whiskey, 1-1/2 ounces. Protein, 5 grams. Carbohydrate, 12 grams. Fat, 7 grams. No glycosuria. Calories, 213.

April 6. Whiskey, 1-1/2 ounces. Protein, 26 grams. Carbohydrate, 18 grams. Fat, 46 grams. No glycosuria. Calories, 768.

April 8. Whiskey, 1-1/2 ounces. Protein, 45 grams. Carbohydrate, 22 grams. Fat, 72 grams. No glycosuria. Calories, 1050.

April 9. Whiskey, 1-1/2 ounces. Protein, 58 grams. Carbohydrate, 36 grams. Fat, 86 grams. No glycosuria. Calories, 1309.

From this her diet was raised gradually until on April 16 she took the following:

Bacon, 4 slices. Oatmeal, 2 tablespoonfuls. Bread, 2 slices. Meat, 1 ounce. Cabbage, 5 tablespoonfuls. Spinach, 5 tablespoonfuls. String beans, 5 tablespoonfuls. Butter, 2 ounces.

This calculated to,

Protein, 64 grams. Carbohydrate, 63 grams. Fat, 113 grams. Calories, 1546. On this diet she excreted .40% sugar.

The next day the bread was cut down to one slice, and her sugar disappeared. On April 20 she was taking 4 tablespoonfuls of oatmeal and one slice of bread with her meat and vegetables, and was sugar-free. This diet contained:

Protein, 63 grams. Carbohydrate, 59 grams. Fat, 112 grams. Calories, 1521.

On April 21, on the same diet, she excreted 1.1% sugar. The next day her oatmeal was cut to 2 tablespoons, giving her about 10 grams less carbohydrate. No glycosuria. She was discharged April 24, sugar-free on

Protein, 63 grams. Carbohydrate, 50 grams. Fat, 112 grams. Calories, 1510.

There had never been any diacetic acid in her urine, and only a trace of acetone. She lost about 2 pounds during starvation, but gained part of it back again, so that at the discharge she weighed just a pound less than when she entered the hospital. She has been reporting to the Out-patient Department every two weeks, and has never had any sugar, acetone or diacetic acid in the urine, and appears to be in splendid condition. She is taking just about the same diet as when she left the hospital.

A rather mild case, which responded readily to treatment. The question is, can she grow and develop on a diet which will keep her sugar-free?

* * * * *

Case 9. M. D., female, age 3-1/2 years, entered April 7, 1915, with a history of having progressively lost weight for a month past, and of having had a tremendous thirst and polyuria. Had been on a general diet at home. At entrance the child was in semi-coma, with very strong sugar, diacetic acid and acetone reactions in the urine. For the first 12 hours she was put on a milk diet, with soda bicarbonate gr. xxx every two hours, and the next day was starved, with whiskey 1 drachm every 2 hours, and soda bicarbonate, both by mouth and rectum. She died after one day of starvation. This is hardly a fair test case of the starvation treatment, as the child was already in coma and almost moribund when she entered the hospital. When a diabetic, old or young, goes into coma, he rarely comes out of it, no matter what the treatment is.

* * * * *

Case 10. H. S., male, 6 years, entered April 29, 1915. Duration of his diabetes uncertain; not discovered until day of entrance. An emaciated, frail looking boy. He would eat very little at first, and on ward diet, containing 31 grams of protein, 73 grams of carbohydrate, and 20 grams of fat, he excreted 5.7% of sugar, with a moderate amount of acetone, and a very slight trace of diacetic acid.

May 2 he was starved, taking 1-1/2 ounces of whiskey. One day of starvation was enough to make him sugar-free. His diet was gradually raised, until on May 7 he was taking 32 grams protein, 33 grams carbohydrate, and 75 grams fat, and was sugar-free, with absent diacetic acid and acetone. May 9 his carbohydrate intake was raised to 45 grams and he excreted .40% sugar. May 10 it was cut to 40 grams, and he excreted 2.2% sugar.

May 11 it was cut to 20 grams, and he became sugar-free and remained so until June 8, when he was discharged, taking the following diet:

String beans, 3 tablespoonfuls. Spinach, 4 tablespoonfuls. Bacon, 4 slices. Butter, 2 ounces. Eggs, 3. Bread, 1/2 slice. Cereal, 2 tablespoonfuls. Meat, 3 ounces. Protein, 63 grams. Carbohydrate, 31 grams. Fat, 113 grams. Calories, 1402.

For the first few days after entrance he showed a moderate amount of acetone and a slight amount of diacetic acid in the urine; for the rest of his stay in the hospital these were absent. His weight at entrance was 31-1/2 pounds; he lost no weight during starvation, and weighed 32-1/2 pounds on discharge.

He was kept on approximately the same diet, and was followed in the Out-patient Department, and on two occasions only did his urine contain a small trace of sugar and of acetone (July 31 and Oct. 16, 1915). Nov. 9 his mother brought him in, saying he had lost his appetite, which had previously been good. The appearance of the boy was not greatly different than it had been all along, but his mother was advised to have him enter the wards immediately, so that he could be watched carefully for a few days. She refused to leave him, but said she would bring him in to stay the next day. She took him home, and he suddenly went into coma and died that night. This was a most unfortunate ending to what seemed to be a very satisfactory case. The boy's mother was an extremely careful and intelligent woman, and it is certain that all directions as to diet were carried out faithfully.

He had never shown any evidence of a severe acidosis, but he must have developed one very suddenly.

* * * * *

Case 11. V. D., 11 years, female, was admitted to the Children's Hospital Nov. 3, 1915. She had had diabetes for at least a year. On house diet, containing about 90 grams of carbohydrate, she excreted 6.9% of sugar, with moderate acetone and diacetic acid reactions in the urine.

Starting Nov. 5, she was starved 3 days. The first day of starvation the sugar dropped to 3.5%, the second day to 1.1%, and the third day she was sugar-free with a little more acetone in the urine than had been present before, but not quite so much diacetic acid. From then her diet was raised as follows:

Nov. 8. Protein, 9 grams. Carbohydrate, 20 grams. Fat, 9 grams. No glycosuria. Calories, 200.

Nov. 9. Protein, 7 grams. Carbohydrate, 15 grams. Fat, 35 grams. No glycosuria. Calories, 415.

Nov. 10. Protein, 17 grams. Carbohydrate, 15 grams. Fat, 55 grams. No glycosuria. Calories, 625.

Nov. 11. Protein, 38 grams. Carbohydrate, 20 grams. No glycosuria. Fat, 88 grams. Calories, 1055.

Nov. 13 two tablespoonfuls of oatmeal were added to her diet, making the carbohydrate intake about 30 grams. This day she showed .6% sugar. She was starved for half a day and became sugar-free again.

On Nov. 16 she was taking protein 40, carbohydrate 20, fat 90, calories 1080, and had no glycosuria.

Nov. 17 her diet was protein 43, carbohydrate 25, fat 140, calories 1538, and on this diet she showed .5% sugar. The carbohydrate was cut to 15 grams, and kept at this level for 3 days, but she still continued to excrete a trace of sugar, and so on Nov. 21 she was starved again, immediately becoming sugar-free. From this her diet was raised, until on discharge, Nov. 30, she was taking: protein 48, carbohydrate 15, fat 110, calories 1280, and was sugar-free, having been so for 9 days.

At entrance she weighed 56 pounds, at discharge 54, and lost 4 pounds during starvation, part of which she gained back again. On the diet which she was taking at discharge, she was just about holding her weight. She never excreted much acetone or diacetic acid, and when she was discharged there was merely the faintest traces of these in the urine.

It is not well to raise the diet quite so rapidly as was done in this case, but for special reasons she had to leave the hospital as soon as possible, and so her diets were pushed up a little faster than would ordinarily be the case.

Below is a graphic chart, such as we use in recording our cases. It has been split up into several pieces here on account of its size:

[Illustration: Case 8. A chart tracking Urine and Calorie Intake for the month of April.]

[Illustration: A chart tracking Carbohydrate and Protein Intake for the month of April.]

[Illustration: A chart tracking per cent. of sugar for the month of April.]

[Illustration: A chart tracking sugar output for the month of April.]

[Illustration: A chart tracking ammonia for the month of April.]

[Illustration: A chart tracking acetone and diacetic acid for the month of April.]

[Illustration: A chart tracking weight in pounds for the month of April.]

EXAMINATION OF THE URINE.

Directions for Collecting Twenty-four Hour Urine.

Pass the urine at 7 a.m. and throw it away.

Save all the urine passed after this up to 7 a.m. the next day. Pass the urine exactly at 7 a.m., and add it to what has previously been passed.

Qualitative Sugar Tests.

(1) Fehling's Test:--Boil about 4 c.c. of Fehling's[1] solution in a test tube, and add to the hot Fehling's an equal amount of urine, a few drops at a time, boiling after each addition.

A yellow or red precipitate indicates sugar.

For practical purposes in the following of a diabetic's daily urine, this is a valuable test, and the one which we always use.

(2) Benedict's Test:--To 5 c.c. of Benedict's[2] reagent add 8 drops of the urine to be examined. The fluid is boiled from 1 to 2 minutes and then allowed to cool of itself. If dextrose is present there results a red, yellow, or green precipitate, depending upon the amount of sugar present. If no sugar is present the solution may remain perfectly clear or be slightly turbid, due to precipitated urates.

This is a more delicate test than Fehling's.

[1] Fehling's solution is prepared as follows:

(a) Copper sulphate solution: 84.65 gm. of copper sulphate dissolved in water and made up to 500 c.c.

(b) Alkaline tartrate solution: 125 gm. of potassium hydroxide and 178 gm. of Rochelle salt dissolved in water and made up to 500 c.c.

These solutions are kept in separate bottles and mixed in equal volumes when ready for use.

[2] Benedict's solution has the following composition:

Copper sulphate, 17.8 gm. Sodium citrate, 178.0 gm. Sodium carbonate (anhydrous), 100 gm. Distilled water to 1000 c.c.

Quantitative Sugar Tests.

(1) The Fermentation Test:--The fermentation test is the simplest quantitative test for sugar, and is quite accurate enough for clinical work. It is performed as follows: The specific gravity of the 24?urine is taken, and 100 c.c. of it put into a flask, and a quarter of a yeast cake crumbled up and added to it. The flask is then put in a warm place (at about body temperature) and allowed to remain over night. The next morning a sample of the fermented urine is tested for sugar. If no sugar is present the urine is made up to 100 c.c. (to allow for the water that has evaporated) and the specific gravity taken again. The number of points loss in specific gravity is multiplied by .23, and this gives the percentage of sugar in the urine.

(2) Benedict's Test:--The best quantitative test for dextrose (excepting polariscopic examination, which is too complicated for ordinary work) is Benedict's test.

It is performed as follows: Measure with a pipette 25 c.c. of Benedict's solution into a porcelain dish, add 5 or 10 gm. (approximately) of solid sodic carbonate, heat to boiling, and while boiling, run in the urine until a white precipitate forms.

Then add the urine more slowly until the last trace of blue disappears. The urine should be diluted so that not less than 10 c.c. will be required to give the amount of sugar which the 25 c.c. of reagent is capable of oxidizing.

Calculation: 5, divided by the number of c.c. of urine run in, equals the per cent. of sugar.

Benedict's quantitative solution is prepared as follows: Dissolve 9.0 gm. of copper sulphate in 100 c.c. distilled water. (The copper sulphate must be weighed very accurately.) Dissolve 50 gm. anhydrous sodic carbonate, 100 gm. sodic citrate, and 65 gm. of potassium sulpho cyanate in 250 c.c. of distilled water.

Pour the copper solution slowly into the alkaline citrate solution. Then pour the mixed solution into the flask without loss, and make up to 500 c.c.; 25 c.c. of this solution is reduced by 50 mgm. of dextrose, 52 mgm. of levulose or 67 mgm. of lactose.

(3) Acetone Test:--To 5 c.c. of urine in a test tube add a crystal of sodium nitro prusside. Acidify with glacial acetic acid, shake a moment, and then make alkaline with ammonium hydrate. A purple color indicates acetone.

(4) Diacetic Acid Test:--To 5 c.c. of urine in a test tube add an excess of a 10% solution of Ferric chloride. A Burgundy red color indicates diacetic acid.

Quantitative Test for Ammonia.

To 25 c.c. of urine add 5 c.c. of a saturated solution of potassium oxalate and 2 to 3 drops of phenolphthalein.

Run in from a burette decinormal sodic hydrate, to a faint pink color. Then add 5 c.c. of formalin (40% commercial) and again titrate to the same color.

Each c.c. of the decinormal alkali used in this last titration equals 1 c.c. of n/10 ammonia, or .0017 gm. of ammonia. Multiply this by the number of c.c. n/10 sodic hydrate used in the last titration; this gives the number of grams of ammonia in 25 c.c. urine.

Note:--The potassium oxalate and the formalin must both be neutral to phenolphthalein.

1 kilogram = 2.2 pounds. 1 calorie = The amount of heat necessary to raise the temperature of 1 kilogram of water 1 degree Centigrade. 1 gram fat = 9.3 calories. 1 gram protein = 4.1 calories. 1 gram carbohydrate = 4.1 calories.

DIETS.

In the diet tables following, the vegetables listed, excepting lettuce, cucumbers, celery, and raw tomatoes, are boiled. In the very low carbohydrate diets they are thrice boiled. When possible to obtain the figures, the analyses for boiled vegetables have been used. It has been estimated that four-tenths of the carbohydrate will go into solution when such vegetables as carrots and cabbage are cut into small pieces, and thoroughly boiled, with changes of water. It must be remembered that bacon loses about half its fat content when moderately cooked.

A number of more or less palatable breads may be made for diabetics, but the majority of the so-called "gluten" and "diabetic flours" are gross frauds, often containing as much as fifty or sixty per cent. carbohydrate. Gluten flour is made by washing away the starch from wheat flour, leaving a residue which is rich in the vegetable protein gluten, so it must be remembered that if it is desired to greatly restrict the protein intake, any gluten flour, even if it contains only a small percentage of carbohydrate, must be used with caution. The report of 1913, Connecticut Agricultural Experiment Station,

Part I, Section 1, "Diabetic Foods", gives a most valuable compilation of

analyses of food products for diabetics. We have found some use for soya meal, casoid flour and Lyster's flour, "akoll" biscuits, and "proto-puffs," but generally the high protein content of all of these foods interferes with giving any large quantity of them to a severe diabetic over a long period of time. The flours mentioned below we know to be reliable.

Some recipes which we have found useful are given below. The use of bran is meant to dilute the protein, increase the bulk, and incidentally to aid in preventing or correcting constipation.

BRAN AND LYSTER FLOUR MUFFINS.[3]

2 level tablespoons lard 2 eggs 4 tablespoons heavy cream, 40% fat 2 cups washed bran 1 package Lyster flour 1/2 cup water or less

Tie dry bran in cheesecloth and soak 1 hour. Wash, by squeezing water through and through, change water several times. Wring dry.

Separate eggs and beat thoroughly. Add to the egg yolks the melted lard, cream and 2 beaten egg whites. Add the Lyster flour, washed bran and water.

Make eighteen muffins.

Total food value: Protein 99 grams, fat 68 grams, carbohydrate 2 grams, calories 1049.

One muffin = protein 5 grams, fat 4 grams, carbohydrate, trace, calories 58.

[3] Lyster's Diabetic Flour prepared by Lyster Brothers, Andover, Mass.

BRAN CAKES.

2 cups wheat bran 2 tablespoons melted butter 2 whole eggs 1 egg white 1/2 teaspoon salt 1/2 grain saccharine

Tie bran in a piece of cheesecloth and soak for one hour. Wash by squeezing water through and through. Change water several times. Wring dry. Dissolve saccharine in one-half teaspoon water. Beat the whole eggs. Mix the bran, beaten eggs, melted butter, and saccharine together. Whip the remaining egg white and fold in at the last. Form into small cakes, using a knife and a tablespoon. Bake on a greased baking sheet until golden brown.

This mixture will make about 25 small cakes. One cake represents 16 calories. A sample cake made by this recipe was analyzed and found to contain neither starch nor sugar.

SOYA MEAL AND BRAN MUFFINS.[4]

1 ounce (30 grams) soya meal 1 level tablespoon (15 grams) butter 1 ounce (30 c.c.) 40% cream 1 cup of washed bran (see method given elsewhere) 1 egg white 1 whole egg may be substituted for 1 egg white 1/4 teaspoon salt 1-1/2 teaspoons baking powder

Mix soya meal, salt and baking powder. Add to the washed bran. Add melted butter and cream. Beat egg white and fold into mixture. Add enough water to make a very thick drop batter. Bake in six well-greased muffin tins until golden brown--from fifteen to twenty-five minutes.

Total food value:

Protein, 11 grams, Fat, 27 grams. Carbohydrate, 2 grams. Calories, 304. One muffin = protein, 2 grams; fat, 4.5 grams. Carbohydrate, trace. Calories, 50.

[4] Soya Bean Meal, Theodore Metcalf Co., Boston, Mass.

CASOID FLOUR AND BRAN MUFFINS.[5]

1 ounce (30 grams) Casoid flour 1 level tablespoon (15 grams) butter 1 ounce (30 c.c.) 40% cream 1 egg white 1 whole egg may be substituted for 1 egg white 1/4 teaspoon salt 1-1/2 teaspoons baking powder 1 cup washed bran

Method as in previous rule. Bake in six muffin tins.

Total food value:

Protein, 18 grams. Fat, 24 grams. Carbohydrate, 1 gram. Calories, 300. One muffin = Protein, 3 grams. Fat, 4 grams. Carbohydrate + Calories, 50.

[5] Casoid Diabetic Flour. Thos. Leeming & Co., Importers, New York City.

LYSTER FLOUR AND BRAN MUFFINS[6]

1 ounce (30 grams) Lyster flour 1 level tablespoon (15 grams) butter 1 ounce (30 c.c.) 40% cream 1 egg white 1 whole egg may be substituted for 1 egg white 1/8 teaspoon salt 1 teaspoon baking powder 1 cup washed bran

Method as in previous recipe. Bake in six muffin tins.

Total food value:

Protein, 18 grams. Fat, 25 grams. Carbohydrate, 1 gram. Calories, 310. One muffin = Protein, 3 grams. Fat, 4 grams. Carbohydrate, trace. Calories, 50.

In order to guard against a monotonous diet, some recipes for special dishes suitable for diabetics are given, most of which can be used in the diets of moderate caloric value. They are taken from "Food and Cookery for the Sick and Convalescent" by Fannie Merritt Farmer.

[6] Lyster's Diabetic Flour prepared by Lyster Brothers. Andover, Mass. Barker's Gluten Flour, Herman Barker, Somerville, Mass.

Note.--In the three preceding recipes one whole egg may be substituted for one egg white. The food value will be slightly increased but the texture of the finished article is improved.

RECIPES.

BUTTERED EGG.

Put one teaspoon butter into a small omelet pan. As soon as the butter is melted break one egg into a cup and slip into the pan. Sprinkle with salt and pepper and cook until white is firm, turning once during the cooking. Care must be taken not to break the yolk.

EGGS AU BEURRE NOIR.

Put one teaspoon butter into a small omelet pan. As soon as butter is melted, break one egg into a cup and slip into the pan. Sprinkle with salt and pepper and cook until white is firm, turning once during the cooking. Care must be taken not to break the yolk. Remove to hot serving dish. In same pan melt one-half tablespoon butter and cook until brown, then add one-fourth teaspoon vinegar. Pour over egg.

EGG ?LA SUISSE.

Heat a small omelet pan and place in it a buttered muffin ring. Put in one-fourth teaspoon butter, and when melted add one tablespoon cream. Break an egg into a cup, slip it into muffin ring, and cook until white is set, then remove ring and put cream by teaspoonfuls over the egg until the cooking is accomplished. When nearly done sprinkle with salt, pepper, and one-half tablespoon grated cheese. Remove egg to hot serving dish and pour over cream remaining in pan.

DROPPED EGG.

Butter a muffin ring, and put it in an iron frying-pan of hot water to which one-half tablespoon salt has been added. Break egg into saucer, then slip into ring allowing water to cover egg. Cover and set on back of range. Let stand until egg white is of jelly-like consistency. Take up ring and egg, using a buttered griddle-cake turner, place on serving dish. Remove ring and garnish egg with parsley.

DROPPED EGG WITH TOMATO PUR 蒙.

Serve a dropped egg with one tablespoon tomato pur 閑. For tomato pur 閑, stew and strain tomatoes, then let simmer until reduced to a thick consistency, and season with salt and pepper and a few drops vinegar. A grating of horseradish root may be added.

EGG FARCI I.

Cut one "hard boiled" egg into halves crosswise. Remove yolk and rub through a sieve. Clean one-half of a chicken's liver, finely chop and saut?in just enough butter to prevent burning. While cooking add a few drops of onion juice. Add to egg yolk, season with salt, pepper, and one-fourth teaspoon finely chopped parsley. Refill whites with mixture, cover with grated cheese, bake until cheese melts. Serve with one tablespoon tomato pur 閑.

EGG FARCI II.

Prepare one egg as for Egg Farci I. Add to yolk one-half tablespoon grated cheese, one-fourth teaspoon vinegar, few grains mustard, and salt and cayenne to taste; then add enough melted butter to make of right consistency to shape. Make into balls the size of the original yolks and refill whites. Arrange on serving-dish, place in a pan of hot water, cover, and let stand until thoroughly heated. Insert a small piece of parsley in each yolk.

BAKED EGG IN TOMATO.

Cut a slice from stem end of a medium-sized tomato, and scoop out pulp. Slip an egg into cavity thus made, sprinkle with salt and pepper, replace cover, put in a small baking pan, and bake until egg is firm.

STEAMED EGG.

Spread an individual earthen mould generously with butter. Season two tablespoons chopped cooked chicken, veal, or lamb, with one-fourth teaspoon salt and a few grains pepper. Line buttered mould with meat and slip in one egg. Cook in a moderate oven until egg is firm. Turn from mould and garnish with parsley.

CHICKEN SOUP WITH BEEF EXTRACT.

1/2 cup chicken stock 1/2 teaspoon Sauterne 1/8 teaspoon beef extract 1-1/2 tablespoons cream Salt and pepper

Heat stock to boiling point and add remaining ingredients.

CHICKEN SOUP WITH EGG CUSTARD.

Serve Chicken Soup with Egg Custard.

Egg Custard.--Beat yolk of one egg slightly, add one-half tablespoon, each, cream and water, and season with salt. Pour into a small buttered tin mould, place in pan of hot water, and bake until firm; cool, remove from mould, cut into fancy shapes.

CHICKEN SOUP WITH EGG BALLS I OR II.

Egg Balls I.--Rub yolk of one hard boiled egg through a sieve, season with salt and pepper, and add enough raw egg yolk to make of right consistency to shape. Form into small balls, and poach in soup.

Egg Balls II.--Rub one-half yolk of hard boiled egg through a sieve, add one-half of a hard boiled egg white finely chopped. Season with salt and moisten with yolk of raw egg until of right consistency to shape. Form and poach same as Egg Balls I.

CHICKEN SOUP WITH ROYAL CUSTARD.

Serve Chicken Soup with Royal Custard.

Royal Custard.--Beat yolk of one egg slightly, add two tablespoons chicken stock, season with salt and pepper, turn into a small buttered mould, and bake in a pan of hot water until firm. Cool, remove from mould, and cut into small cubes or fancy shapes.

ONION SOUP.

Cook one-half large onion, thinly sliced, in one tablespoon butter eight minutes. Add three-fourths cup chicken stock, and let simmer twenty minutes. Rub through a sieve, add two tablespoons cream, and yolk one-half egg beaten slightly. Season with salt and pepper.

ASPARAGUS SOUP.

12 stalks asparagus, or 1/3 cup canned asparagus tips 2/3 cup chicken stock 1/4 slice onion. Yolk one egg 1 tablespoon heavy cream 1/8 teaspoon salt Few grains pepper

Cover asparagus with cold water, bring to boiling point, drain, and add stock and onion; let simmer eight minutes, rub through a sieve, reheat, add cream, egg and seasonings. Strain and serve.

TOMATO BISQUE.

2/3 cup canned tomatoes 1/4 slice onion Bit of bay leaf 2 cloves 1/4 cup boiling water 1/8 teaspoon soda 1/2 tablespoon butter 1/4 teaspoon salt Few grains pepper 2 tablespoons heavy cream

Cook first five ingredients for eight minutes. Rub through sieve, add soda, butter in small pieces, seasoning, and cream. Serve at once.

CAULIFLOWER SOUP.

1/3 cup cooked cauliflower 2/3 cup chicken stock Small stalk celery 1/4 slice onion 1 egg yolk 1 tablespoon heavy cream 2 teaspoons butter Salt and pepper

Cook cauliflower stalk, celery and onion eight minutes. Rub through pur 閑 strainer, reheat, add egg yolk slightly beaten, cream, butter, and seasoning.

MUSHROOM SOUP.

3 mushrooms 2/3 cup chicken stock 1/4 slice onion 2 teaspoons butter 1 egg yolk 1 tablespoon heavy cream 1 teaspoon sauterne Salt and pepper

Clean mushrooms, chop, and cook in one teaspoon butter five minutes. Add stock and let simmer eight minutes. Rub through a pur 閑 strainer, add egg yolk slightly beaten, cream, remaining butter, seasoning and wine.

SPINACH SOUP.

1 tablespoon cooked chopped spinach 2/3 cup chicken stock 1 egg yolk 1 tablespoon heavy cream Salt and pepper

Cook spinach with stock eight minutes. Rub through a pur 閑 strainer, reheat, add egg yolk slightly beaten, cream, and seasoning.

BROILED FISH, CUCUMBER SAUCE.

Serve a small piece of broiled halibut, salmon, or sword fish, with cucumber sauce.

Cucumber Sauce.--Pare one-half cucumber, grate and drain. Season with salt, pepper and vinegar.

BAKED FILLET OF HALIBUT, HOLLANDAISE SAUCE.

Wipe a small fillet of halibut and fasten with a skewer. Sprinkle with salt and pepper, place in pan, cover with buttered paper and bake twelve minutes. Serve with,

Hollandaise Sauce.--Put yolk of one egg, one tablespoon butter, and one teaspoon lemon juice in a small sauce-pan. Put sauce-pan in a larger one containing water, and stir mixture constantly with wooden spoon until butter is melted. Then add one-half tablespoon butter, and as the mixture thickens another one-half tablespoon butter; season with salt and cayenne. This sauce is almost thick enough to hold its shape. One-eighth teaspoon of beef extract, or one-third teaspoon grated horseradish added to the first mixture gives variety to this sauce.

BAKED HALIBUT WITH TOMATO SAUCE.

Wipe a small piece of halibut, and sprinkle with salt and pepper. Put in a buttered pan, cover with a thin strip of fat salt pork gashed several times, and bake twelve to fifteen minutes. Remove fish to serving dish, discarding pork. Cook eight minutes one-third cup of tomatoes, one-fourth slice onion, one clove, and a few grains salt and pepper. Remove onion and clove and run through a sieve. Add a few grains soda and cook until tomato is reduced to two teaspoons. Pour around fish and garnish with parsley.

HALIBUT WITH CHEESE.

Sprinkle a small fillet of halibut with salt and pepper, brush over with melted butter, place in pan and bake twelve minutes. Remove to serving dish and pour over it the following sauce:

Heat two tablespoons cream, add one-half egg yolk slightly beaten, and when well mixed one tablespoon grated cheese. Season with salt and paprika.

FINNAN HADDIE ?LA DELMONICO.

Cover a small piece of finnan haddie with cold water, place on back of range and allow water to heat gradually to boiling point, then keep below boiling point for twenty minutes. Drain, rinse thoroughly, and separate into flakes; there should be two tablespoons. Reheat over hot water with one hard boiled egg thinly sliced in two tablespoons heavy cream. Season with salt and paprika, add one teaspoon butter and sprinkle with finely chopped parsley.

FILLET OF HADDOCK WITH WINE SAUCE.

Remove skin from a small piece of haddock, put in a buttered baking pan, pour over it one teaspoon melted butter, one tablespoon white wine, and a few drops, each, of lemon juice and onion juice. Cover and bake. Remove to serving dish, and to liquor in pan add one tablespoon cream and one egg yolk slightly beaten. Season with salt and pepper. Strain over fish, and sprinkle with finely chopped parsley.

SMELTS WITH CREAM SAUCE.

Clean two selected smelts and cut five diagonal gashes on sides of each. Season with salt, pepper, and lemon juice. Cover and let stand ten minutes. Roll in cream, dip in flour, and saut?in butter. Remove to serving dish, and to fat in pan add two tablespoons cream. Cook three minutes, season with salt, pepper, and a few drops lemon juice. Strain sauce around smelts and sprinkle with finely chopped parsley.

SMELTS ?LA MA 螩 RE D'HOTEL.

Prepare smelts same as for smelts with cream, and serve with ma 頪 re d'hotel butter.

SALT CODFISH WITH CREAM.

Pick salt codfish into flakes; there should be two tablespoons. Cover with lukewarm water and let stand on back of range until soft. Drain, and add three tablespoons cream; as soon as cream is heated add yolk one small egg slightly beaten.

SALT CODFISH WITH CHEESE.

To salt codfish with cream, add one-half tablespoon grated cheese and a few grains paprika.

BROILED BEEFSTEAK, SAUCE FIGARO.

Serve a portion of broiled beefsteak with Sauce Figaro.

Sauce Figaro.--To Hollandaise sauce add one teaspoon tomato pur 閑. To prepare tomato pur 閑 stew tomatoes, force through a strainer and cook until reduced to a thick pulp.

ROAST BEEF, HORSERADISH CREAM SAUCE.

Serve a slice of rare roast beef with Horseradish Cream Sauce.

Horseradish Cream Sauce.--Beat one tablespoon heavy cream until stiff. As cream begins to thicken, add gradually three-fourths teaspoon vinegar. Season with salt and pepper, then fold in one-half tablespoon grated horseradish root.

FILLET OF BEEF.

Wipe off a thick slice cut from tenderloin. Put in hot frying pan with three tablespoons butter. Sear one side, turn and sear other side. Cook eight minutes, turning frequently, taking care that the entire surface is seared, thus preventing the escape of the inner juices.

Remove to hot serving dish, and pour over fat in pan, first strained through cheesecloth. Garnish with cooked cauliflower, canned string beans, reheated and seasoned, and saut 閑 mushroom caps.

LAMB CHOPS, SAUCE FINESTE.

Serve lamb chops with Sauce Fineste.

Sauce Fineste.--Cook one-half tablespoon butter until browned. Add a few grains, each, mustard and cayenne, one-fourth teaspoon Worcestershire Sauce, and a few drops lemon juice, and two tablespoons stewed and strained tomatoes.

SPINACH.

Chop one cup cooked spinach drained as dry as possible. Season with salt and pepper, press through a pur 閑 strainer, reheat in butter, using as much as desired or as much as the spinach will take up. Arrange on serving dish and garnish with white of "hard boiled" egg cut in strips and yolk forced through strainer.

BRUSSELS SPROUTS WITH CURRY SAUCE.

Pick over Brussels sprouts, remove wilted leaves, and soak in cold salt water fifteen minutes. Cook in boiling salted water twenty minutes, or until easily pierced with skewer. Drain, and pour over one-fourth cup curry sauce.

Curry Sauce.--Mix one-fourth teaspoon mustard, one-fourth teaspoon salt, and a few grains paprika. Add yolk of one egg slightly beaten, one tablespoon olive oil, one and one-half tablespoons vinegar, and a few drops of onion juice. Cook over hot water, stirring constantly until mixture thickens. Add one-fourth teaspoon curry powder, one teaspoon melted butter, and one-eighth teaspoon chopped parsley.

FRIED CAULIFLOWER.

Steam or boil a small cauliflower. Cool and separate into pieces. Saut?enough for one serving in olive oil until thoroughly heated. Season with salt and pepper, arrange on serving-dish, and pour over one tablespoon melted butter.

CAULIFLOWER ?LA HUNTINGTON.

Separate hot steamed cauliflower into pieces and pour over sauce made same as sauce for Brussels sprouts with curry sauce.

CAULIFLOWER WITH HOLLANDAISE SAUCE.

Serve boiled cauliflower with Hollandaise sauce, as given with baked fillet of halibut, Hollandaise sauce.

MUSHROOMS IN CREAM.

Clean, peel and break in pieces six medium-sized mushroom caps. Saut?in one-half tablespoon butter three minutes. Add one and one-half tablespoons cream and cook until mushrooms are tender. Season with salt and pepper and a slight grating of nutmeg.

BROILED MUSHROOMS.

Clean mushrooms, remove stems, and place caps on a buttered broiler. Broil five minutes, having gills nearest flame during first half of broiling. Arrange on serving dish, put a small piece of butter in each cap and sprinkle with salt and pepper.

SUPREME OF CHICKEN.

Force breast of uncooked chicken through a meat chopper; there should be one-fourth cup. Add one egg beaten slightly and one-fourth cup heavy cream. Season with salt and pepper. Turn into slightly buttered mould, set in pan of hot water and bake until firm.

SARDINE RELISH.

Melt one tablespoon butter, and add two tablespoons cream. Heat to boiling point, add three sardines freed from skin and bones, and separated in small pieces, and one hard-boiled egg finely chopped. Season with salt and cayenne.

DIABETIC RAREBIT.

Beat two eggs slightly and add one-fourth teaspoon salt, a few grains cayenne, and two tablespoons, each, cream and water. Cook same as scrambled eggs, and just before serving add one-fourth Neufch铋el cheese mashed with fork.

CHEESE SANDWICHES.

Cream one-third tablespoon butter and add one-half tablespoon, each, finely chopped cold boiled ham and cold boiled chicken; then season with salt and paprika. Spread between slices of Gruy鐩e cheese cut as thin as possible.

CHEESE CUSTARD.

Beat one egg slightly, add one-fourth cup cold water, two tablespoons heavy cream, one tablespoon melted butter, one tablespoon grated cheese and a few grains salt. Turn into an individual mould, set in pan of hot water, and bake until firm.

COLD SLAW.

Select a small heavy cabbage, remove outside leaves, and cut cabbage in quarters; with a sharp knife slice very thinly. Soak in cold water until crisp; drain, dry between towels, and mix with cream salad dressing.

CABBAGE SALAD.

Finely shred one-fourth of a small firm cabbage. Let stand two hours in salted cold water, allowing one tablespoon of salt to a pint of water. Cook slowly thirty minutes one-fourth cup, each, vinegar and cold water, with a bit of bay leaf, one-fourth teaspoon peppercorns, one-eighth teaspoon mustard seed and three cloves. Strain and pour over cabbage drained from salted water. Let stand two hours, again drain, and serve with or without mayonnaise dressing.

CABBAGE AND CELERY SALAD.

Wash and scrape two stalks of celery, add an equal quantity of shredded cabbage, and six walnut meats broken in pieces. Serve with cream dressing.

CUCUMBER CUP.

Pare a cucumber and cut in quarters cross wise. Remove center from one piece and fill cup thus made with tartare sauce. Serve on lettuce leaf.

CUCUMBER AND LEEK SALAD.

Cut cucumber in small cubes and leeks in very thin slices. Mix, using equal parts, and serve with French dressing.

CUCUMBER AND WATERCRESS SALAD.

Cut cucumbers in very thin slices, and with a three-tined fork make incisions around the edge of each slice. Arrange on a bed of watercress.

EGG SALAD I.

Cut one hard-boiled egg in halves crosswise, in such a way that tops of halves may be left in points. Remove yolk, mash, moisten with cream, French or mayonnaise dressing, shape in balls, refill whites, and serve on lettuce leaves. Garnish with thin slices of radish, and a radish so cut as to represent a tulip.

EGG SALAD.

Prepare egg same as for Egg Salad I, adding to yolk an equal amount of chopped cooked chicken or veal.

EGG AND CHEESE SALAD.

Prepare egg same as for Egg Salad I, adding to yolk three-fourths tablespoon grated cheese; season with salt, cayenne and a few grains of mustard; then moisten with vinegar and melted butter. Serve with or without salad dressing.

EGG AND CUCUMBER SALAD.

Cut one hard boiled egg in thin slices. Cut as many very thin slices from a chilled cucumber as there are slices of egg. Arrange in the form of a circle (alternating egg and cucumber), having slices overlap each other. Fill in center with chicory or watercress. Serve with salad dressing.

CHEESE SALAD.

Mash one-sixth of a Neufch 鉳 el cheese and moisten with cream. Shape in forms the size of a robin's egg. Arrange on a lettuce leaf and sprinkle with finely chopped parsley which has been dried. Serve with salad dressing.

CHEESE AND OLIVE SALAD.

Mash one-eighth of a cream cheese, and season with salt and cayenne. Add finely chopped olives, two lettuce leaves, finely cut, and a small piece of canned pimento, to give color. Press in original shape of cheese and let stand two hours. Cut in slices and serve on lettuce leaves with mayonnaise dressing.

CHEESE AND TOMATO SALAD.

Peel and chill one medium-sized tomato, and scoop out a small portion of the pulp. Mix equal quantities of Roquefort and Neufch 鉳 el cheese and mash, then moisten with French dressing. Fill cavity made in tomato with cheese. Serve on lettuce leaves with French dressing.

FISH SALAD I.

Remove salmon from can, rinse thoroughly with hot water and separate in flakes; there should be one-fourth cup. Mix one-eighth teaspoon salt, a few grains, each, mustard and paprika, one teaspoon melted butter, one-half tablespoon cream, one tablespoon water, one-half tablespoon vinegar and yolk of one egg; cook over hot water until mixture thickens; then add one-fourth teaspoon granulated gelatin soaked in one teaspoon cold water. Add to salmon, mould, chill, and serve with cucumber sauce.

Cucumber Sauce.--Pare one-fourth cucumber; chop, drain, and add French dressing to taste.

ASPARAGUS SALAD.

Drain and rinse four stalks of canned asparagus. Cut a ring one-third inch wide from a red pepper. Put asparagus stalks through ring, arrange on lettuce leaves, and pour over French dressing.

TOMATO JELLY SALAD.

Season one-fourth cup hot stewed and strained tomato with salt, and add one-third teaspoon granulated gelatin soaked in a teaspoon cold water. Turn into an individual mould, chill, turn from mould, arrange on lettuce leaves, and garnish with mayonnaise dressing.

FROZEN TOMATO SALAD.

Season stewed and strained tomato with salt and cayenne. Fill a small tin box with mixture, cover with buttered paper, then tight-fitting cover, pack in salt and ice, equal parts, and let stand two hours. Remove from mould, place on lettuce leaf and serve with mayonnaise dressing.

TOMATO JELLY SALAD WITH VEGETABLES.

Cook one-third cup tomatoes with bay leaf, sprig of parsley, one-sixth slice onion, four peppercorns, one clove, eight minutes. Remove vegetables and rub tomato through a sieve; there should be one-fourth cup. Add one-eighth teaspoon granulated gelatin soaked in one teaspoon cold water, a few grains salt, and four drops vinegar. Line an individual mould with cucumber cut in fancy shapes, and string beans, then pour in mixture. Chill, remove from mould, arrange on lettuce leaf, and garnish with mayonnaise dressing.

TOMATO BASKET OF PLENTY.

Cut a medium-sized tomato in shape of a basket, leaving stem end on top of handle. Fill basket with cold cooked string beans cut in small pieces and two halves of English walnut meats cut in pieces, moistened with French dressing. Serve on lettuce leaf.

TOMATO AND CHIVE SALAD.

Remove skin from small tomato. Chill and cut in halves crosswise. Spread with mayonnaise, sprinkle with finely chopped chives, and serve on lettuce leaf.

CANARY SALAD.

Cut a slice from the stem end of a bright red apple and scoop out pulp, leaving enough to keep shell in shape. Fill shell thus made with grapefruit pulp and finely chopped celery, using twice as much grapefruit as celery. It will be necessary to drain some of the juice from the grapefruit. Moisten with mayonnaise dressing, replace the cover and arrange on lettuce leaf, and garnish with a canary made from Neufch 鉳 el cheese, coloring yellow and shaping, designating eyes with paprika and putting a few grains on the body of the bird. Also garnish with three eggs made from cheese, colored green and speckled with paprika.

Note.--Do not use apple pulp.

HARVARD SALAD.

Cut a selected lemon in the form of a basket with handle, and scoop out all the pulp. Fill basket thus made with one tablespoon cold cooked chicken or sweet bread cut in small dice, mixed with one-half tablespoon small cucumber dice, and one teaspoon finely chopped celery moistened with cream or mayonnaise dressing. Spread top with dressing and sprinkle with thin parings cut from round red radishes finely chopped. Insert a small piece of parsley on top of handle. Arrange on watercress.

CUCUMBER BOATS.

Cut a small cucumber in halves lengthwise. Scoop out centres and cut boat-shaped. Cut cucumber cut from boats in small pieces and add one and one-half olives finely chopped. Moisten with French dressing, fill boats with mixture and serve on lettuce leaves.

SPINACH SALAD.

Drain and finely chop one-fourth cup cooked spinach. Season with salt, pepper, lemon juice, and melted butter. Pack solidly in an individual mould, chill, remove from mould, and arrange on a thin slice of cooked tongue cut in circular shape. Garnish base of mould with wreath of parsley and top with sauce tartare.

Sauce Tartare.--To one tablespoon mayonnaise dressing add three-fourths teaspoon finely chopped capers, pickles, olives, and parsley, having equal parts of each.

SWEETBREAD AND CUCUMBER SALAD.

Mix two tablespoons cold cooked sweetbread cut in cubes, one tablespoon cucumber cubes, and one-half tablespoon finely chopped celery. Beat one and one-half tablespoons heavy cream until stiff, then add one-eighth teaspoon granulated gelatin dissolved in one teaspoon boiling water and three-fourths teaspoon vinegar. Set in a pan of ice water and as mixture begins to thicken, add sweetbreads and vegetables. Mould and chill. Remove from mould, arrange on lettuce leaves, and garnish top with a slice of cucumbers and sprig of parsley.

CHICKEN AND NUT SALAD.

Mix two tablespoons cold cooked chicken or fowl cut in cubes with one tablespoon finely chopped celery and one-half tablespoon English walnut meats browned in oven with one-eighth teaspoon butter and a few grains salt, then broken in pieces. Moisten with mayonnaise dressing. Mound and garnish with curled celery, tips of celery, and whole nut meats.

PRINCESS PUDDING

1 egg yolk 3/4 teaspoon granulated gelatin dissolved in 1 tablespoon boiling water 2 teaspoons lemon juice 1/4 grain saccharine dissolved in 1/4 teaspoon cold water 1 egg white.

Beat egg yolk until thick and lemon-colored, add gelatin, continue the beating. As mixture thickens add gradually the lemon juice and saccharine. Fold in white of egg beaten until stiff and dry. Turn into a mould and chill.

COFFEE BAVARIAN CREAM.

2 tablespoons coffee infusion 1 tablespoon water 2 tablespoons heavy cream 1 egg yolk Few grains salt 3/4 teaspoon granulated gelatin soaked in 1 teaspoon cold water. 1 grain saccharine dissolved in 1/2 teaspoon cold water 1 egg white 1/4 teaspoon vanilla

Scald coffee, water and one-half cream. Add egg yolk, slightly beaten, and cook until mixture thickens; then add gelatin and salt. Remove from fire, cool, add saccharine, remaining cream beaten stiff, egg white beaten until stiff, and teaspoon vanilla. Turn into mould and chill.

LEMON CREAM SHERBET.

1/4 cup cream 2 tablespoons cold water 1/2 grain saccharine dissolved in 1/2 teaspoon cold water 4 drops lemon juice Few grains salt

Mix ingredients in order given and freeze.

ORANGE ICE.

1/3 cup orange juice 1 teaspoon lemon juice 2 tablespoons cold water 1/2 grain saccharine dissolved in 1/2 teaspoon cold water

Mix ingredients in order given, and freeze.

GRAPEFRUIT ICE.

1/4 cup grapefruit juice 1/4 cup water 1/2 grain saccharine dissolved in 1/2 teaspoon cold water.

Remove juice from grapefruit, strain and add remaining ingredients, and freeze to a mush. Serve in sections of grapefruit.

FROZEN PUNCH.

1/4 cup cream 2 tablespoons cold water 1-1/2 teaspoons rum 1 egg yolk 1/2 grain saccharine dissolved in 1/2 teaspoon cold water Few grains salt

Scald one-half cream with water, add egg yolk slightly beaten and cook over hot water until mixture thickens. Cool, add remaining ingredients and freeze.

DIET LISTS.

Attention is called to the fact that the protein allowance in the following diets is not large. The first two tables represent fast days; the next six are transitional days, in which the nourishment is gradually increased but does not satisfy the caloric needs. The remainder may be selected according to the needs of the case or the weight of the patient.

To prevent monotony or to give variety, one meat may be substituted for another, or one "5%" vegetable for another. The fat may be increased by the addition of butter or olive oil if more calories are needed to maintain body weight. However, it is not considered desirable to give so much fat that the weight will increase.

TABLE I.

Protein, 10 grams Carbohydrate, 15 grams Fat, 7 grams Calories, 200

BREAKFAST. String beans (canned). 120 grams 2-1/2 h. tbsp. Asparagus (canned). 150 grams 3 h. tbsp. or 13-1/2 stalks 4 in. long. Tea or coffee.

DINNER. Celery. 100 grams 6 pieces 4-1/2 in. long. Spinach (cooked). 135 grams 3 h. tbsp. Tea or coffee.

SUPPER. Asparagus. 100 grams 2 h. tbsp. or 9 stalks 4 in. long. Celery. 100 grams 6 pieces 4-1/2 in. long. Tea or coffee.

TABLE II.

Protein, 7 grams Carbohydrate, 15 grams Fat, 6 grams Calories, 150

BREAKFAST. Asparagus (canned). 75 grams 1-3/4 h. tbsp. (chopped). Cabbage. 65 grams 1 very h. tbsp. Tea or coffee.

DINNER. Onions (cooked). 100 grams 2 h. tbsp. Celery. 50 grams 3 pieces about 4-1/2 in. long. Tea or coffee.

SUPPER. Spinach. 100 grams 2 h. tbsp. Celery. 50 grams 3 pieces 4-1/2 in. long. Tea or coffee.

TABLE III.

Protein, 24 grams Carbohydrate, 8 grams Fat, 22 grams Calories, 340

BREAKFAST. String beans. 100 grams 2 h. tbsp. Egg. 1 Coffee.

DINNER. Egg. 1 Turnips. 100 grams 2 h. tbsp. Cabbage. 100 grams 2 h. tbsp. Tea.

SUPPER. Egg. 1 Turnips. 100 grams 2 h. tbsp. Spinach. 100 grams 2 h. tbsp. Tea.

TABLE IV.

Protein, 31 grams Fat, 14 grams Carbohydrate, 17 grams Calories, 327

BREAKFAST. Egg. 1 Asparagus. 100 grams 2 h. tbsp. Tomatoes. 100 grams 2 h. tbsp. Coffee.

DINNER. Chicken. 35 grams 1 small serving. String beans. 200 grams 4 h. tbsp. Cabbage. 100 grams 2 h. tbsp. Tea or coffee.

SUPPER. Egg. 1 Cauliflower. 240 grams 5 h. tbsp. + Spinach. 100 grams 2 h. tbsp. Tea or coffee.

TABLE V.

Protein, 43 grams Carbohydrate, 15 grams Fat, 19 grams Calories, 414

BREAKFAST. Egg. 1 Asparagus. 200 grams 4 h. tbsp. Coffee.

DINNER. Chicken. 70 grams 1 mod. serving. Cauliflower. 120 grams 2 h. tbsp.

Cabbage (cooked). 100 grams 2 h. tbsp. Tea.

SUPPER. Egg. 1 String beans. 100 grams 2 h. tbsp. Spinach. 200 grams 4 h. tbsp. Tea.

TABLE VI.

Protein, 38 grams Fat, 31 grams Carbohydrate, 19 grams Calories, 520

BREAKFAST. Egg. 1 Asparagus. 200 grams 4 h. tbsp. Coffee.

DINNER. Steak. 100 grams 1 small serving. Celery (cooked). 200 grams 4 h. tbsp. Tea.

SUPPER. Egg. 1 Lettuce. 20 grams 2 medium leaves. Cucumbers. 100 grams 2 h. tbsp. String beans. 50 grams 1 h. tbsp. Tea.

TABLE VII.

Protein, 35 grams Carbohydrate, 17 grams Fat, 100 grams Calories, 1143

BREAKFAST. Bacon. 50 grams 2 slices about 6 in. long. Asparagus. 100 grams 2 h. tbsp. or 9 stalks 4 in. long (canned). Spinach. 100 grams 2 h. tbsp. Butter. Cream. Coffee.

DINNER. Steak. 100 grams 1 small serving. Turnips. 140 grams 2 h. tbsp. + Spinach. 100 grams 2 h. tbsp. Cabbage. 100 grams 2 h. tbsp. Butter. Tea. Cream.

SUPPER. Spinach. 100 grams 2 h. tbsp. String beans (cooked). 100 grams 2 h. tbsp. Cauliflower (cooked). 120 grams 2 h. tbsp. + Butter. Tea. Cream.

Allow during day: Butter. 20 grams 2 squares. Cream, 40%. 2-1/2 ounces 5 tbsp.

TABLE VIII.

Protein, 40 grams Carbohydrate, 16 grams Fat, 104 grams Calories, 1196

BREAKFAST. Egg. 1 Asparagus. 100 grams 2 h. tbsp or 9 stalks 4 in. long (canned). Spinach. 100 grams 2 h. tbsp. Butter. Coffee. Cream.

DINNER. Steak. 100 grams 1 small serving. Turnips. 140 grams 2 h. tbsp. + Celery. 100 grams 2 h. tbsp. Cabbage. 100 grams 2 h. tbsp. Butter. Cream. Tea.

SUPPER. Bacon. 50 grams 2 slices about 6 in. long. Spinach. 100 grams 2 h. tbsp. String beans (canned). 100 grams 2 h. tbsp. Cauliflower. 100 grams 2 h. tbsp. Butter. Cream. Tea.

Allow during day: Butter. 20 grams 2 squares. Cream 40%. 3 ounces 6 tbsp.

TABLE IX.

Protein, 50 grams Carbohydrate, 15 grams Fat, 125 grams Calories, 1500

BREAKFAST. Eggs. 2 String beans(canned). 100 grams 3 h. tbsp. Butter. Cream. Coffee.

DINNER. Chop. 100 grams 1 chop. Cabbage (cooked). 100 grams 2 h. tbsp. Cucumbers. 100 grams 2 h. tbsp. Tea. Butter. Cream.

SUPPER. Egg. 1 Asparagus (canned). 100 grams 2 h. tbsp. Cauliflower (cooked). 100 grams 2 h. tbsp. Butter. Cream. Tea.

Allow during day: Butter. 25 grams 2-1/2 square. Cream, 40%. 5 ounces 10 tbsp.

TABLE X.

Protein, 61 grams Carbohydrate, 16 grams Fat, 160 grams Calories, 1795

BREAKFAST. Bacon. 50 grams 2 slices 6 in. long. Eggs. 2 Spinach. 100 grams 2 h. tbsp. Butter. Cream. Coffee.

DINNER. Steak. 100 grams 1 small serving. Tomatoes (canned). 100 grams 2 h. tbsp. Butter. Cream. Tea.

SUPPER. Chicken. 50 grams 1 small serving. Lettuce. 20 grams 2 leaves. Celery. 100 grams 6 stalks 4-1/2 in. long. Butter. Cream. Tea.

Allow during day: Butter. 50 grams 5 squares. Cream, 40%. 5 ounces 10 tbsp.

TABLE XI.

Protein, 38 grams Carbohydrate, 20 grams Fat, 100 grams Calories 1168

BREAKFAST. Bacon. 30 grams 1-1/2 slices 6 in. long. Egg. 1 Spinach. 100 grams 2 h. tbsp. Coffee. Butter. Cream.

DINNER. Steak. 50 grams 1 very small serving. Cabbage. 100 grams 2 h. tbsp. Onions. 100 grams 2 h. tbsp. Butter. Cream. Tea.

SUPPER. Scraped beef balls. 40 grams = 1-1/3 oz. Chopped celery salad. 100 grams 2 h. tbsp. Tomatoes. 100 grams 2 tbsp.

Allow during day: Butter. 25 grams 2-1/2 squares. Cream, 40%. 4 ounces 8 tbsp.

TABLE XII.

Protein, 35 grams Carbohydrate, 16 grams Fat, 92 grams Calories, 1064

BREAKFAST. Egg. 1 Cabbage. 100 grams 2 h. tbsp. Tomatoes. 100 grams 2 h. tbsp. Butter. Coffee. Cream.

DINNER. Steak. 80 grams 1 small serving. Spinach. 100 grams 2 h. tbsp. Turnips. 140 grams 2 h. tbsp. + Egg, white. 1 Butter. Cream. Tea.

SUPPER. Cauliflower. 120 grams 2 h. tbsp. + Onions. 100 grams 2 h. tbsp. Lettuce. 10 grams 1 leaf. Olive oil. 5 grams 1 teaspoon. + Tea. Butter. Cream.

Allow during day: Butter. 25 grams 2-1/2 squares. Cream, 40%. 3 ounces 6 tbsp.

TABLE XIII.

Protein, 40 grams Fat, 110 grams Carbohydrate, 21 grams Calories, 1187

BREAKFAST. Bacon. 50 grams 2 slices 6 in. long. Cauliflower. 120 grams 2 h. tbsp. Butter. Cream. Coffee.

DINNER. Squab. 1 Carrots. 100 grams 2 h. tbsp. Tomatoes. 100 grams 2 h. tbsp. Butter. Cream. Tea.

SUPPER. Turnips. 140 grams 2 h. tbsp. + Asparagus. 100 grams 2 h. tbsp. Celery. 100 grams 6 stalks 4-1/2 in. long. Butter. Cream. Tea.

Allow during day: Butter. 20 grams 2 squares. Cream, 40%. 3-1/2 ounces 7 tbsp.

TABLE XIV.

Protein, 40 grams Carbohydrate, 20 grams Fat, 103 grams Calories, 1200

BREAKFAST. Egg. 1 + 1 egg white. Spinach. 200 grams 4 h. tbsp. Cream. Butter.

DINNER. Steak. 50 grams 1 very small serving. Cabbage. 100 grams 2 h. tbsp. Tomatoes. 100 grams 2 h. tbsp. Onions. 100 grams 2 h. tbsp. Butter. Cream. Tea.

SUPPER. Scraped beef balls 40 grams 1-1/3 oz. Celery. 100 grams 6 stalks 4-1/2 in. long. Cream. Butter. Tea.

Allow during day: Butter. 20 grams 2 squares. Cream, 40%. 5 ounces 10 tbsp.

TABLE XV.

Protein, 40 grams Carbohydrate, 22 grams Fat, 105 grams Calories, 2100

BREAKFAST. Egg. 1 Asparagus. 100 grams 2 h. tbsp. Butter. Cream. Coffee.

DINNER. Chop. 105 grams 1 medium. Peas. 50 grams 1 h. tbsp. Celery. 50 grams 6 stalks 4-1/2 in. long. Butter. Cream. Tea.

SUPPER. Cauliflower. 120 grams 2 h. tbsp. + String beans. 100 grams 2 h. tbsp. Butter. Cream. Tea.

Allow during day: Butter. 20 grams 2 squares. Cream, 40%. 4 ounces 8 tbsp.

TABLE XVI.

Protein 40 grams Fat, 100 grams Carbohydrate, 30 grams Calories, 1200

BREAKFAST. Bacon. 50 grams 2 slices 6 in. long. Peas (canned). 75 grams 1-3/4 h. tbsp. Butter. Cream. Coffee.

DINNER. Broth--6 ounces with vegetables: Cabbage. 25 grams 1 level tbsp. Tomatoes. 25 grams 1 level tbsp. Turnips. 25 grams 1 level tbsp. Celery. 50 grams 3 pieces 4-1/2 in. long. Steak. 100 grams 1 small serving. Squash. 50 grams 1 h. tbsp. Tomatoes. 75 grams 1-3/4 tbsp. Butter. Cream. Tea.

SUPPER. Spinach. 100 grams 2 h. tbsp. Turnips. 175 grams 3-3/4 h. tbsp. Celery. 100 grams 6 stalks 4-1/2 in. long.

Allow during day: Butter. 50 grams 5 squares. Cream, 40%. 4 ounces 8 tbsp.

TABLE XVII.

Protein, 40 grams Carbohydrate, 30 grams Fat, 100 grams Calories, 1200

BREAKFAST. Bacon. 50 grams 2 slices about 6 in. long. Egg. 1 Asparagus (chopped). 100 grams 2 h. tbsp. Butter. Cream. Coffee.

DINNER. Chicken. 50 grams 1 small serving. Cabbage. 100 grams 2 h. tbsp. Cauliflower. 120 grams 2 h. tbsp. + Cucumbers. 100 grams 2 h. tbsp. Butter. Cream. Tea.

SUPPER. Turnips. 140 grams 2 h. tbsp. String beans. 100 grams 2 h. tbsp. Bread. 25 grams 1 thin slice, baker's loaf. Butter. Cream. Tea.

Allow during day: Butter. 25 grams 2-1/2 squares. Cream, 40%. 4 ounces 8 tbsp.

TABLE XVIII.

Protein, 40 grams Carbohydrate, 35 grams Fat, 110 grams Calories, 1330

BREAKFAST. Bacon. 50 grams 2 slices about 6 in. long. Peas. 75 grams 1-3/4 h. tbsp. Tomatoes. 100 grams 2 h. tbsp. Butter. Cream. Coffee.

DINNER. Broth--chicken, lamb or beef. 6 ounces Steak. 100 grams 1 small serving. Turnips. 200 grams 4 h. tbsp. Celery. 150 grams 9 stalks 4-1/2 in. long. Butter. Cream. Tea.

SUPPER. Squash. 50 grams 1 h. tbsp. Beets. 100 grams 2 h. tbsp. Cabbage (raw). 25 grams 1 h. tbsp. Butter. Cream. Tea.

Allow during day: Butter. 25 grams 2-1/2 squares. Cream, 40%. 4 ounces 8 tbsp.

TABLE XIX.

Protein, 40 grams Carbohydrate, 35 grams Fat, 115 grams Calories, 1370

BREAKFAST. Bacon. 50 grams 3 slices 6 in. long. Parsnips. 100 grams 2 h. tbsp. Potatoes (boiled). 50 grams 1 very small one. Butter. Cream. Coffee.

DINNER. Broth. 6 ounces Squab. 1 Cabbage. 100 grams 2 h. tbsp. Celery 100 grams 6 stalks about 4-1/2 in. long. Butter. Cream. Tea.

SUPPER. String beans. 140 grams 3 h. tbsp. Cucumbers. 100 grams 2 h. tbsp. Parsnips. 100 grams 2 h. tbsp. Cauliflower. 120 grams 2 h. tbsp. + Milk. 4 ounces 1/2 glass. Butter. Cream. Tea.

Allow during day: Butter. 20 grams 2 squares. Cream, 40%. 4 ounces 8 tbsp.

TABLE XX.

Protein, 50 grams Carbohydrate, 35 grams Fat, 130 grams Calories, 1557

BREAKFAST. Orange. 100 grams 1 small. Bacon. 50 grams 3 slices, 6 in. long. Egg. 1 Spinach. 100 grams 2 h. tbsp. Butter. Cream. Coffee.

DINNER. Broth. 180 c.c. 1 glass or cup. Steak. 100 grams 1 small serving. Boiled onions. 100 grams 2 h. tbsp. Butter. Cream. Tea.

SUPPER. Egg. 1 Lettuce. 25 grams 3 small leaves. Bread. 20 grams 1 very thin slice. Cream. Tea. Butter.

Allow during day: Butter. 25 grams 2-1/2 squares. Cream, 40%. 4 ounces 8 tbsp.

TABLE XXI.

Protein, 50 grams Carbohydrate, 40 grams Fat, 158 grams Calories, 1830

BREAKFAST. Bacon. 50 grams 2 slices 6 in. long. Bread. 20 grams 1 slice, 3 x 3 x 1/2 in. Spinach. 100 grams 2 h. tbsp. Butter. Cream. Coffee.

DINNER. Broth. 180 c.c. 1 glass or cup. Steak. 100 grams 1 small serving. Cabbage. 100 grams 2 h. tbsp. Lettuce. 100 grams 10 leaves. Butter. Cream. Tea.

SUPPER. Egg. 1 Onions (boiled). 100 grams 2 h. tbsp. Bread. 15 grams 1 slice very thin, 3 x 3 x 1/4 Milk. 4 ounces 8 tbsp. Butter. Cream. Tea.

Allow during day: Butter. 50 grams 5 squares. Cream, 40%. 5 ounces 10 tbsp.

TABLE XXII.

Protein, 60 grams Carbohydrate, 30 grams Fat, 158 grams Calories, 1830

BREAKFAST. Bacon. 50 grams 2 slices 6 in. long. Egg. 1 Tomatoes. 100 grams 2 h. tbsp. Cream. Butter. Coffee.

DINNER. Steak. 100 grams 1 small serving. Turnips. 420 grams 4 h. tbsp. + Cucumbers. 100 grams 2 h. tbsp. Onions. 100 grams 2 medium sized. Butter. Cream. Tea. Olive oil. 21 grams 1-1/2 tbsp.

SUPPER. Chicken. 50 grams 1 small serving. Lettuce. 100 grams 10 medium leaves. Celery. 100 grams 6 stalks 4-1/2 in. long. Spinach. 100 grams 2 h. tbsp. Butter. Tea. Cream.

Allow during day: Butter. 15 grams 1-1/2 squares. Cream, 40%. 6 ounces 12 tbsp.

TABLE XXIII.

Protein, 62 grams Carbohydrate, 31 grams Fat, 153 grams Calories, 1800

BREAKFAST. Bacon. 50 grams 2 slices. Peas. 75 grams 1-1/2 h. tbsp. Butter. Cream. Coffee.

DINNER. Broth--100 c.c. with vegetables: = 7 tbsp. Cabbage. 25 grams 1 level tbsp. Tomato. 25 grams 1 level tbsp. Turnip. 25 grams 1 level tbsp. Celery (chopped). 50 grams 2 level tbsp. Steak. 100 grams 1 small serving. Squash. 50 grams 1 h. tbsp. Tomatoes. 75 grams 1-1/2 h. tbsp. Butter. Cream. Tea.

SUPPER. Chicken. 75 grams 1 small serving. Turnips. 175 grams 2-3/4 h. tbsp. Celery. 100 grams 6 stalks 4-1/2 in. long.

Allow during day: Butter. 50 grams 5 squares. Cream, 40%. 5 ounces 10 tbsp. Olive oil. 7 grams 1/? tbsp. +

TABLE XXIV.

Protein, 60 grams Carbohydrate, 30 grams Fat, 158 grams Calories, 1830

BREAKFAST. Bacon. 50 grams 2 slices 6 in. long. Egg. 1 Turnips. 140 grams 3 h. tbsp. -- Butter. Cream. Coffee.

DINNER. Steak. 100 grams 1 small serving. Celery. 100 grams 6 stalks 4-1/2 in. long. Cucumbers. 100 grams 2 h. tbsp. Lettuce. 100 grams 10 leaves.

Spinach. 100 grams 2 h. tbsp. Olive oil. 21 grams 1-1/2 tbsp. + Butter. Cream. Tea.

SUPPER. Chicken. 50 grams 1 very small serving. Turnips. 280 grams 4 h. tbsp. + Onions. 100 grams 2 h. tbsp. Tomatoes. 100 grams 2 h. tbsp. Butter. Cream. Tea.

Allow during day: Butter. 50 grams 5 squares. Cream, 40%. 5 ounces 10 tbsp.

TABLE XXV.

Protein, 60 grams Carbohydrate, 30 grams Fat, 154 grams Calories, 1800

BREAKFAST. Bacon. 60 grams 2-1/2 slices, 6 in. long. Eggs. 2 Turnips. 140 grams 2-1/2 h. tbsp.

DINNER. Steak. 100 grams 1 small serving. Spinach. 50 grams 1 h. tbsp. Parsnips. 150 grams 3 h. tbsp. Onions. 100 grams 2 h. tbsp. Beets. 50 grams 1 h. tbsp. Butter. Cream. Tea.

SUPPER. Ham. 50 grams 1 very small serving. Lettuce. 100 grams 10 leaves. String beans. 50 grams 1 h. tbsp. Celery. 100 grams 6 stalks 4-1/2 in. long. Asparagus. 50 grams 1 h. tbsp.

Allow during day: Butter. 40 grams 4 squares. Cream, 40%. 4 ounces 8 tbsp.

TABLE XXVI.

Protein, 40 grams Carbohydrate, 36 grams Fat, 105 grams Calories, 1280

BREAKFAST. Bacon. 50 grams 2 slices. Parsnips. 100 grams 2 h. tbsp. Potatoes (mashed). 60 grams 1 h. tbsp. Butter. Cream. Coffee.

DINNER. Broth. 180 c.c. 1 glass. Squab. 100 grams 1 squab (small). Cabbage. 100 grams 2 tbsp. Celery. 100 grams 6 stalks 4-1/2 in. long. Butter. Cream. Tea.

SUPPER. String beans. 100 grams 2 h. tbsp. Cucumbers. 100 grams 2 h. tbsp.

Parsnips. 100 grams 2 h. tbsp. Cauliflower. 120 c.c. 2 h. tbsp. + Milk. 120 c.c. 1/2 glass. Butter. Cream. Tea.

Allow during day: Butter. 20 grams 2 squares. Cream, 40%. 4 ounces 8 tbsp.

TABLE XXVII.

Protein, 50 grams Carbohydrate, 40 grams Fat, 131 grams Calories, 1587

BREAKFAST. Egg. 1 Parsnips. 100 grams 2 h. tbsp. Bread. 35 grams 1 slice, 3 x 3-1/2 x 1/2 in. Butter. Cream. Coffee.

DINNER. Broth. 180 c.c. 1 glass or cup. Chop. 100 grams 1 Cauliflower. 120 grams 2 h. tbsp. + Carrots. 100 grams 2 h. tbsp. Butter. Cream. Tea.

SUPPER. Bacon. 50 grams 2 slices. Lettuce. 25 grams 3 leaves. String beans. 100 grams 2 h. tbsp. Peas. 55 grams 1 h. tbsp. + Spinach. 100 grams 2 h. tbsp. Butter. Cream. Tea.

Allow during day: Butter. 25 grams 2-1/2 squares. Cream, 40%. 3 ounces 6 tbsp.

TABLE XXVIII.

Protein, 50 grams Carbohydrate, 50 grams Fat, 124 grams Calories, 1563

BREAKFAST. Orange. 100 grams 1 small. Eggs. 2 Bread. 10 grams 1 slice, 2 x 1 x 1/2 in. Butter. Cream. Coffee.

DINNER. Steak. 100 grams 1 small serving. Lettuce. 100 grams 10 leaves. Spinach. 100 grams 2 h. tbsp. Butter. Cream. Tea.

SUPPER. Egg. 1 Cold ham. 50 grams 1 small serving. Asparagus. 50 grams 1 h. tbsp. String beans. 100 grams 2 h. tbsp. Bread. 25 grams 1 slice, 3 x 3 x 1/2 in. Butter. Cream. Tea.

Allow during day: Butter. 30 grams 3 squares. Cream, 40%. 4 ounces 8 tbsp.

TABLE XXIX.

Protein, 52 grams Carbohydrate, 52 grams Fat, 116 grams Calories, 1504

BREAKFAST. Orange. 100 grams 1 small. Bacon. 50 grams 2 slices 6 in. long. Egg. 1 Bread. 20 grams 1 slice, 3 x 2 x 1/2 in. Butter. Cream. Coffee.

DINNER. Boiled ham. 100 grams 1 large slice (thin). Brussels sprouts. 100 grams 2 h. tbsp. Milk. 6 ounces 1 glass. Butter. Tea. Cream.

SUPPER. Scotch broth. 6 ounces 12 tbsp. Lettuce. 50 grams 5 leaves. Bread. 20 grams 1 slice, 3 x 2 x 1/2 in.

Allow during day: Butter. 20 grams 2 squares. Cream, 40%. 3 ounces 6 tbsp.

TABLE XXX.

Protein, 50 grams Carbohydrate, 50 grams Fat, 117 grams Calories, 1590

BREAKFAST. Orange. 100 grams 1 small. Bread. 25 grams 1 slice, 3 x 2 x 1/2 in. Egg. 1 Bacon. 50 grams 2 slices 6 in. long. Butter. Cream. Coffee.

DINNER. Chop. 100 grams 1 medium chop. Asparagus. 100 grams 2 h. tbsp. Butter. Cream. Tea.

SUPPER. Egg. 1 Cucumbers. 100 grams 2 h. tbsp. Lettuce. 10 grams 1 leaf. Bread. 25 grams 1 slice, 3 x 2 x 1/2 in.

Allow during day: Butter. 30 grams 3 squares. Cream, 40%. 3 ounces 6 tbsp.

TABLE XXXI.

Protein, 53 grams Carbohydrate, 50 grams Fat, 133 grams Calories, 1658

BREAKFAST. Orange. 150 grams 1 medium. Bacon. 60 grams 2-1/2 slices. Egg. 1 Bread. 20 grams 1 slice, 3 x 2 x 1/2 in. Butter. Cream. Tea.

DINNER. Steak. 50 grams 1 very small serving. String beans. 50 grams 1 h.

tbsp. Lettuce. 100 grams 10 leaves. Butter. Cream. Tea.

SUPPER. Ham. 50 grams 1 small slice. Asparagus. 50 grams 1 h. tbsp. Spinach. 50 grams 1 h. tbsp. Bread. 15 grams 1 slice, 3 x 1 x 1/2 in. Butter. Cream. Tea.

Allow during day: Butter. 20 grams 2 squares. Cream, 40%. 3 ounces 6 tbsp.

TABLE XXXII.

Protein, 101 grams Carbohydrate, 51 grams Fat, 255 grams Calories, 2995

BREAKFAST. Orange. 50 grams 1/2 orange (small). Steak. 100 grams 1 slice. Egg. 1 Bread. 20 grams 1 slice, 3 x 2 x 1/2 in. Butter. Cream. Tea.

DINNER. Lamb chop. 180 grams 2 small. Potato. 50 grams 1 very small. Turnip. 140 grams 2 h. tbsp + Lettuce. 10 grams 1 leaf. Tomato (raw). 100 grams 1 medium. Custard--made with one egg and part of the cream. Butter. Tea. Olive oil. 1-1/2 tbsp.

SUPPER. Bacon. 50 grams 2 slices 6 in. long. Eggs. 2 Onions. 50 grams 1 h. tbsp. Cabbage. 100 grams 2 h. tbsp. Bread. 20 grams 1 slice, 3 x 2 x 1/2 in. Butter. Cream. Tea.

Allow during day: Butter. 50 grams 5 squares. Cream, 40%. 6 ounces 12 tbsp.

TABLE XXXIII.

Protein, 60 grams Carbohydrate, 55 grams Fat, 159 grams Calories, 1950

BREAKFAST. Orange. 100 grams 1 small. Bacon. 100 grams 4 slices 6 in. long. Egg. 1 Spinach. 100 grams 2 h. tbsp. Bread. 25 grams 1 slice, 3 x 2 x 1/2 in. Butter. Cream. Coffee.

DINNER. Broth. 180 c.c. 1 glass or cup. Steak. 100 grams 1 small serving. Parsnips. 100 grams 2 h. tbsp. Carrots. 100 grams 2 h. tbsp. Butter. Cream. Tea.

SUPPER. Egg. 1 Lettuce. 25 grams 3 medium leaves. String beans. 10 grams 2

h. tbsp. Bread. 25 grams 1 slice, 3 x 2 x 1/2 in. Spinach. 60 grams 1 very h. tbsp. Butter. Cream. Tea.

Allow during day: Butter. 25 grams 2-1/2 squares. Cream, 40%. 4 ounces 8 tbsp.

TABLE XXXIV.

Protein, 60 grams Carbohydrate, 50 grams Fat, 145 grams Calories, 1800

BREAKFAST. Egg. 1 Bacon. 100 grams 4 slices 6 in. long. Tomatoes. 100 grams 2 h. tbsp. Bread. 35 grams 1 slice, medium. Butter. Cream. Tea.

DINNER. Broth. 180 c.c. 1 glass or cup. Squab. 100 grams 1 squab (small). Cabbage. 100 grams 2 h. tbsp. Onions. 100 grams 2 h. tbsp. Butter. Cream. Tea.

SUPPER. Egg. 1 Lettuce. 25 grams 3 medium leaves. Celery. 100 grams 6 stalks, 4-1/2 in. long. Bread. 30 grams 1 slice, med. thin.

Allow during day: Butter. 30 grams 3 squares. Cream, 40%. 3-1/2 ounces 7 tbsp.

TABLE XXXV.

Protein, 63 grams Carbohydrate, 60 grams Fat, 140 grams Calories, 1800

BREAKFAST. Grape fruit. 100 grams 1/2 small grape fruit. Bacon. 100 grams 4 slices 6 in. long. Egg. 1 Cauliflower. 120 grams 2 h. tbsp. + Bread. 30 grams 1 slice, med. thin. Butter. Cream. Coffee.

DINNER. Broth. 180 c.c. 1 glass. Squab. 100 grams 1 squab. Carrots. 100 grams 2 h. tbsp. Lettuce. 100 grams 10 leaves. Asparagus. 100 grams 2 h. tbsp. Butter. Cream. Tea.

SUPPER. Egg. 1 Asparagus. 100 grams 2 h. tbsp. Spinach. 100 grams 2 h. tbsp. Bread. 30 grams 1 slice, med. thin. Butter. Cream. Tea.

Allow during day: Butter. 20 grams 2 squares. Cream, 40%. 3 ounces 6 tbsp.

TABLE XXXVI.

Protein, 60 grams Carbohydrate, 60 grams Fat, 140 grams Calories, 1794

BREAKFAST. Orange. 100 grams 1 small. Bacon. 100 grams 4 slices 6 in. long. Egg. 1 Bread. 35 grams 1 slice medium. Butter. Cream. Tea.

DINNER. Broth. 180 c.c. 1 glass or cup. Steak. 100 grams 1 small serving. Turnips. 140 grams 2 h. tbsp. + Parsnips. 200 grams 4 h. tbsp. String beans. 100 grams 2 h. tbsp. Butter. Cream. Tea.

SUPPER. Egg. 1 Lettuce. 25 grams 3 leaves. Cucumbers. 100 grams 16 slices (thin). Bread. 30 grams 1 slice, med. thin. Butter. Cream. Tea.

Allow during day: Butter. 20 grams 2 squares. Cream, 40%. 3 ounces 6 tbsp.

TABLE XXXVII.

Protein, 74 grams Carbohydrate, 62 grams Fat, 179 grams Calories, 2220

BREAKFAST. Bacon. 100 grams 4 slices 6 in. long. Egg. 1 Bread. 30 grams 1 slice, 3 x 3 x 1/2 in. medium thin. Butter. Cream. Tea.

DINNER. Broth. 180 c.c. 1 glass. Chicken. 100 grams 1 medium serving. Baked potato. 100 grams 1 medium. Tomato. 100 grams 2 h. tbsp. Lettuce. 25 grams 3 leaves. Olive oil. 13 grams 1 tbsp. Butter. Cream. Tea.

SUPPER. Egg. 1 Cabbage. 100 grams 2 h. tbsp. Celery. 100 grams 6 stalks 4-1/2 in. long. Onions. 100 grams 2 h. tbsp. Butter. Tea. Cream.

Allow during day: Butter. 25 grams 2-1/2 squares. Cream, 40%. 7 ounces 14 tbsp.

TABLE XXXVIII.

Protein, 71 grams Carbohydrate, 60 grams Fat, 184 grams Calories, 2242

BREAKFAST. Bacon. 100 grams 4 slices 6 in. long Egg. 1 Asparagus. 100 grams 2 h. tbsp. Bread. 25 grams 1 slice, 3 x 2 x 1/2 in. Butter. Cream. Coffee.

DINNER. Broth. 180 c.c. 1 glass or cup. Steak. 100 grams 1 small serving. Spinach. 100 grams 2 h. tbsp. Carrots. 100 grams 2 h. tbsp. Butter. Cream. Tea.

SUPPER. Egg. 1 Lettuce. 100 grams 10 leaves. Lima beans. 100 grams 2 h. tbsp. Cauliflower. 120 grams 2 h. tbsp. + Beef juice. 4 ounces 8 tbsp. Bread. 25 grams 1 slice 3 x 3 x 1/2 in. Butter. Cream. Tea.

Allow during day: Butter. 25 grams 2-1/2 squares. Cream, 40%. 7 ounces 14 tbsp.

TABLE XXXIX.

Protein, 72 grams Carbohydrate, 65 grams Fat, 174 grams Calories, 2170

BREAKFAST. Bacon. 100 grams 4 slices 6 in. long. Eggs. 2 Bread. 25 grams 1 slice, 3 x 2 x 1/2 in. Butter. Cream. Coffee.

DINNER. Broth. 180 c.c. 1 glass or cup. Squab. 100 grams 1 Lettuce. 25 grams 3 leaves. Cucumbers. 100 grams 1 h. tbsp. Turnips. 140 grams 2 h. tbsp. Strawberries. 100 grams 2 h. tbsp. + Bread. 25 grams 1 slice, 3 x 2 x 1/2 in. Butter. Cream. Tea.

SUPPER. Fish (Haddock). 1 very small helping. String beans. 100 grams 2 h. tbsp. Parsnips. 200 grams 4 h. tbsp. Bread. 25 grams 1 slice, 3 x 2 x 1/2 in. Butter. Cream. Tea.

Allow during day: Butter. 10 grams 1 square. Cream, 40%. 7 ounces 14 tbsp.

TABLE XL.

Protein, 71 grams Carbohydrate, 65 grams Fat, 183 grams Calories, 2257

BREAKFAST. Bacon. 100 grams 4 slices 6 in. long. Egg. 1 Bread. 20 grams 1 very small slice. Carrots. 100 grams 2 h. tbsp. Butter. Cream. Coffee.

DINNER. Broth. 180 c.c. 1 glass or cup. Roast lamb. 100 grams 1 small serving. Baked potato. 100 grams 1 medium. Lettuce. 10 leaves. Asparagus. 100 grams 2 h. tbsp. Butter. Cream. Tea.

SUPPER. Eggs. 2 Cauliflower. 120 grams 2 h. tbsp. + Spinach. 100 grams 2 h. tbsp. Bread. 20 grams 1 very small slice. Butter. Cream. Tea.

Allow during day: Butter. 25 grams 2-1/2 squares. Cream, 40%. 7 ounces 14 tbsp.

TABLE XLI.

Protein, 77 grams Carbohydrate, 68 grams Fat, 185 grams Calories, 2315

BREAKFAST. Bacon. 100 grams 4 slices 6 in. long. Eggs. 2 Tomatoes. 100 grams 1 med. tomato. Butter. Cream. Tea.

DINNER. Broth. 6 ounces 1 glass. Haddock. 100 grams 1 small helping. Cabbage. 100 grams 2 h. tbsp. Onions. 100 grams 2 h. tbsp. Baked potato. 100 grams 1 medium. Tea. Cream. Butter.

SUPPER. Cold boiled ham. 75 grams 1 slice, large. Bread. 25 grams 1 slice, 3 x 2 x 1/2 in. Peas. 100 grams 2 h. tbsp. Lettuce. 25 grams 3 leaves. Celery. 100 grams 6 stalks 4-1/2 in. long. Butter. Tea.

Allow during day: Butter. 35 grams 3-1/2 squares. Cream, 40%. 7 ounces 14 tbsp.

TABLE XLII.

Protein, 77 grams Carbohydrate, 69 grams Fat, 186 grams Calories, 2328

BREAKFAST. Bacon. 100 grams 4 slices 6 in. long. Eggs. 2 Bread. 50 grams 2 slices, 3 x 2 x 1/2 in. Butter. Cream. Coffee.

DINNER. Broth. 6 ounces 1 glass or cup. Steak. 100 grams 1 slice. Turnips. 140 grams 2 h. tbsp. + Lettuce. 25 grams 3 leaves. Bread. 25 grams 1 slice, 3 x

2 x 1/2 in. Cream. Tea.

SUPPER. Cold veal. 50 grams 1 small slice. Parsnips. 200 grams 4 h. tbsp. String beans. 100 grams 2 h. tbsp. Cucumbers. 100 grams 2 h. tbsp. Bread. 25 grams 1 slice, 3 x 2 x 1/2 in. Cream. Tea.

Allow during day: Butter. 30 grams 3 squares. Cream, 40%. 7 ounces 14 tbsp.

TABLE XLIII.

Protein, 74 grams Carbohydrate, 71 grams Fat, 176 grams Calories, 2220

BREAKFAST. Egg. 1 Bacon. 100 grams 4 slices 6 in. long. Parsnips. 100 grams 2 h. tbsp. Butter. Cream. Coffee.

DINNER. Broth. 6 ounces 1 glass or cup. Chicken. 100 grams 1 med. serving. Squash. 50 grams 1 h. tbsp. Turnips. 140 grams 2 h. tbsp. + String beans. 100 grams 2 h. tbsp. Baked potato. 100 grams 1 medium. Butter. Cream. Tea.

SUPPER. Egg. 1 Parsnips. 100 grams 2 h. tbsp. Lettuce. 25 grams 3 leaves. Cucumbers. 100 grams 2 h. tbsp. Bread. 40 grams 1 slice, 3 x 2 x 1/2 in. Olive oil. 13 grams 1 tbsp. Butter. Cream. Tea.

Allow during day: Butter. 20 grams 2 squares. Cream, 40%. 7 ounces 14 tbsp.

TABLE XLIV.

Protein, 75 grams Carbohydrate, 71 grams Fat, 180 grams Calories, 2250

BREAKFAST. Bacon. 100 grams 4 slices 6 in. long. Egg. 1 Asparagus. 100 grams 2 h. tbsp. Potato (boiled). 50 grams 1 very small. Butter. Cream. Tea.

DINNER. Steak. 100 grams 1 small serving. Potato (boiled). 100 grams 1 medium. Spinach. 100 grams 2 h. tbsp. Cauliflower. 120 grams 2 h. tbsp. + Butter. Cream. Tea.

SUPPER. Egg. 1 Cottage cheese. 50 grams 1-1/2 x 1-1/2 x 1-1/2 in. Lettuce. 100 grams 10 leaves. Carrots. 100 grams 2 h. tbsp. Bread. 35 grams 1 med.

thin slice. Butter. Cream. Tea.

Allow during day: Butter. 20 grams 2 squares. Cream, 40%. 7 ounces 14 tbsp.

TABLE XLV.

Protein, 99 grams Carbohydrate, 101 grams Fat, 225 grams Calories, 2880

BREAKFAST. Oranges. 200 grams 2 small. Bacon. 75 grams 3 slices. Eggs. 2 Bread. 35 grams 1 med. slice. Butter. Cream. Coffee.

DINNER. Lamb chop. 100 grams 1 chop. Peas. 100 grams 2 h. tbsp. Olives. 50 grams 13 small olives. Almonds. 50 grams 26 small almonds. Bread. 25 grams 1 slice, 3 x 2 x 1/2 in. Butter. Cream. Tea.

SUPPER. Salmon. 100 grams 1 average helping. Salad: Lettuce. 25 grams 3 leaves. Fresh tomato. 100 grams 1 medium. Mayonnaise. 21 grams 1 tbsp. American cheese. 25 grams 1-1/2 x 1 x 1 in. Bread. 40 grams 1 slice, 3 x 3-1/2 x 1/2 in.

Allow during day: Butter. 40 grams 4 squares. Cream, 40%. 6 ounces 12 tbsp.

TABLE XLVI.

Protein, 101 grams Carbohydrate, 101 grams Fat, 235 grams Calories, 3010

BREAKFAST. Grape fruit. 100 grams 1/2 small. Eggs. 2 Bread. 50 grams 2 slices, 3 x 2 x 1/2 in. Butter. Cream. Coffee.

DINNER. Chops. 200 grams 2 small. Potato. 75 grams 1 medium or 1-1/2 tbsp. of mashed. Lettuce. 50 grams 5 leaves. Bread. 25 grams 1 slice, 3 x 2 x 1/2 in. Walnuts. 25 grams 5 whole walnut meats. French dressing: Oil. 26 grams 2 tbsp. Vinegar.

SUPPER. Cold chicken. 50 grams 1 small slice. Egg. 1 Bread. 25 grams 1 slice, 3 x 2 x 1/2 in. Celery. 50 grams 3 stalks 4-1/2 in. long. Peach. 100 grams 1 peach. Butter. Cream. Tea.

Allow during day: Butter. 50 grams 5 squares. Cream, 40%. 6 ounces 12 tbsp.

TABLE XLVII.

Protein, 99 grams Carbohydrate, 126 grams Fat, 228 grams Calories, 3043

BREAKFAST. Lamb chop. 100 grams 1 chop. Eggs. 2 Bread. 50 grams 2 slices, each 3 x 2 x 1/2 in. Butter. Cream. Coffee.

DINNER. Steak. 100 grams 1 small serving. Potato. 200 grams 2 small ones. Cabbage. 100 grams 2 h. tbsp. Bread. 25 grams 1 slice, 3 x 2 x 1/2 in. Butter. Tea. Custard or ice cream, using part of cream, and one-half egg (extra).

SUPPER. Bacon. 100 grams 4 slices. Egg. 1 Peas. 100 grams 2 h. tbsp. Beets. 100 grams 2 h. tbsp. Peach (as purchased). 100 grams 1 peach. Bread. 25 grams 1 slice, 3 x 2 x 1/2 in. Butter. Cream. Tea.

Allow during day: Butter. 50 grams 5 squares. Cream, 40%. 6 ounces 12 tbsp.

TABLE XLVIII.

Protein, 101 grams Carbohydrate, 150 grams Fat, 292 grams Calories, 3744

BREAKFAST. Grape fruit. 300 grams 1 medium. Bacon. 75 grams 3 slices. Eggs. 2 Bread. 35 grams 1 medium slice. Butter. Cream. Tea. Sugar.

DINNER. Lamb chop. 100 grams 1 chop. Peas. 100 grams 2 h. tbsp. Lettuce. 25 grams 3 leaves. Fresh tomato. 100 grams 1 medium. Mayonnaise. 21 grams 1 tbsp. Bread. 25 grams 1 slice, 3 x 2 x 1/2 in. Butter. Tea.

SUPPER. Cold roast beef. 100 grams 1 slice (large). Olives. 50 grams 13 small olives. Almonds. 20 grams Cream cheese. 50 grams 1-1/2 x 1-1/2 x 1-1/2 in. Bread. 40 grams 1 slice, 3 x 3-1/2 x 1/2 in. Butter. Cream. Tea.

Allow during day: Butter. 50 grams 5 squares. Cream, 40%. 5 ounces 10 tbsp. Sugar. 40 grams 4 h. tbsp. Tea. Butter.

* * * * *

Dr. Edwin A. Locke's book of food values has been of much value in making up these diets.

* * * * *

The following shows the successive steps in building up a diet for a patient who starved six days before becoming sugar-free:

Grams Grams Grams Total Protein Fat Carbohydrate Calories

Day 1 2 + 5 30 " 2 15 12 4 189 " 3 23 18 8 294 " 4 36 30 11 471 " 5 18 48 9 560 " 6 51 44 17 688 " 7 52 51 15 750 " 8 46 51 19 740 " 9 49 78 20 1008 " 10 50 101 21 1230 " 11 49 123 19 1422 " 12 Starved because sugar came through " 13 15 12 3 185 " 14 34 32 10 478 " 15 53 100 15 1208

* * * * *

Patient discharged with advice as to diet. The corresponding menus for the above are as follows:

FIRST DAY.

BREAKFAST. DINNER. SUPPER.

String beans 25 grams. Lettuce 25 grams. Lettuce 25 grams. Lettuce 25 grams. Cucumbers 25 grams. Tomato 25 grams. Coffee. Tea. Tea.

Protein 2 grams, Fat, trace, Carbohydrate 5 grams, Calories 30.

SECOND DAY.

BREAKFAST. DINNER. SUPPER.

Egg 1. Egg 1. Lettuce 25 grams. Lettuce 25 grams. Lettuce 25 grams. String beans 25 grams. Cucumbers 25 grams. String beans 25 grams. Tea. Coffee. Tea.

Protein 15 grams, Fat 12 grams, Carbohydrate 4 grams, Calories 189.

THIRD DAY.

BREAKFAST. DINNER. SUPPER.

Egg 1. Egg 1. Egg 1. Asparagus 50 grams. Cauliflower 50 grams. String beans 75 grams. Lettuce 25 grams. Lettuce 50 grams. Celery 50 grams.

Protein 28 grams, Fat 18 grams, Carbohydrate 8 grams, Calories 294.

FOURTH DAY.

BREAKFAST. DINNER. SUPPER.

Egg 1. Chicken broth 6 oz. Egg 1. String beans 100 grams. Egg 1. Egg whites 2. Coffee. Celery 100 grams. Lettuce 75 grams. Cream 1 oz. Tea. Cucumbers 50 grams.

Protein 36 grams, Fat 30 grams, Carbohydrate 11 grams, Calories 471.

FIFTH DAY.

BREAKFAST. DINNER. SUPPER.

Egg 1. String beans 75 grams. Egg 1. Cauliflower 100 grams. Lettuce 25 grams. Asparagus. Coffee. Tomatoes 50 grams. Tea. Cream 2 tbsp. Butter 1 square. Cream 2 tbsp. Butter 1/2 square. Tea. Cream 2 tbsp.

Protein 18 grams, Fat 48 grams, Carbohydrate 10 grams, Calories 560.

SIXTH DAY.

BREAKFAST. DINNER. SUPPER.

Egg 1. Broth 6 oz. Egg 1. Spinach 75 grams. Chicken 50 grams. Egg whites 2. Butter 1/2 square. Lettuce 50 grams. String beans 75 grams. Coffee. Tomatoes 75 grams. Cucumbers 75 grams. Cream 1 tbsp. Asparagus 75 grams.

Tea. Tea. Cream 1 tbsp. Cream 1 tbsp. Butter 1/2 square.

Protein 51 grams, Fat 44 grams, Carbohydrate 17 grams, Calories 688.

SEVENTH DAY.

BREAKFAST. DINNER. SUPPER.

Eggs 2. Beef broth 6 oz. Egg 1. Asparagus 100 grams. Scraped beef 50 grams. Salmon 50 grams. Coffee. Cauliflower 100 grams. Cabbage 100 grams. Cream 1 tbsp. Spinach 100 grams. Tomatoes (raw) 75 grams. Lettuce 25 grams. String beans 100 grams. Tea. Tea. Cream 1 tbsp. Cream 1 tbsp.

Protein 52 grams, Fat 51 grams, Carbohydrate 15 grams, Calories 750.

EIGHTH DAY.

BREAKFAST. DINNER. SUPPER.

Egg 1. Chicken 75 grams. Egg 1. String beans 100 grams. Cauliflower 100 grams. Spinach 100 grams. Asparagus 100 grams. Olives 25 grams. Celery 50 grams. Coffee. Cucumbers 50 grams. Lettuce 50 grams. Cream 1 tbsp. Tea. Tea. Cream 1 tbsp. Cream 1 tbsp.

Protein 46 grams, Fat 51 grams, Carbohydrate 19 grams, Calories 740.

NINTH DAY.

BREAKFAST. DINNER. SUPPER.

Egg 1. Chicken 75 grams. Egg 1. Egg white 1. String beans 100 grams. Cauliflower 100 grams. Spinach 100 grams. Asparagus 100 grams. Cucumbers 50 grams. Celery 50 grams. Olives 25 grams. Lettuce 50 grams. Coffee. Tea. Tea. Cream 2 tbsp. Cream 1 tbsp. Cream 1 tbsp. Butter 1 square. Butter 1-1/2 square. Butter 1 square.

Protein 49 grams, Fat 77 grams, Carbohydrate 19 grams, Calories 1008.

TENTH DAY.

BREAKFAST. DINNER. SUPPER.

Egg 1. Lamb chop 75 grams. Egg 1. Lettuce 50 grams. Spinach 100 grams. Salmon 50 grams. String beans 100 grams. Celery 50 grams. Asparagus 100 grams. Cucumbers 100 grams. Olives 25 grams. Cabbage 100 grams. Coffee. Tea. Tea. Cream 2 tbsp. Cream 2 tbsp. Cream 2 tbsp.

Protein 50 grams, Fat 101 grams, Carbohydrate 21 grams, Calories 1230.

ELEVENTH DAY.

BREAKFAST. DINNER. SUPPER.

Bacon 50 grams. Beef broth 8 oz. Egg 1. Asparagus 100 grams. Chicken 75 grams. Tomatoes 100 grams. Spinach 100 grams. Cabbage 100 grams. Spinach 50 grams. Butter 2 squares. Cucumbers 50 grams. Butter 2 squares. Cream 3 tbsp. Butter 3 squares. Cream 1 tbsp. Cream (made into ice cream) 4 tbsp.

Protein 49 grams, Fat 123 grams, Carbohydrate 19 grams, Calories 1422.

TWELFTH DAY.

BREAKFAST. DINNER. SUPPER.

Black coffee. Chicken broth 8 oz. Beef broth 8 oz.

Protein 12 grams, Calories 49.

THIRTEENTH DAY.

BREAKFAST. DINNER. SUPPER.

String beans 50 grams. Egg 1. Egg 1. Black coffee. Asparagus 50 grams. Cabbage 50 grams. Tea. Tea.

Protein 15 grams, Fat 12 grams, Carbohydrate 4 grams, Calories 185.

FOURTEENTH DAY.

BREAKFAST. DINNER. SUPPER.

Egg 1. Roast chicken 50 grams. Egg 1. String beans 100 grams. Asparagus 100 grams. Cauliflower 100 grams. Coffee. Cabbage 100 grams. Tea. Cream 1 tbsp. Tea. Cream 1 tbsp. Cream 1 tbsp.

Protein 34 grams, Fat 32 grams, Carbohydrate 10 grams, Calories 478.

FIFTEENTH DAY.

BREAKFAST. DINNER. SUPPER.

Egg 1. Squab 100 grams. Egg 1. Tomatoes 50 grams. String beans 100 grams. Cold chicken 25 grams. Coffee. Cauliflower 150 grams. Lettuce 50 grams. Cream 2 tbsp. Butter 1 square. Spinach 50 grams. Custard made with 1 Tea. egg, 4 tbsp. cream Cream 2 tbsp. and 2 tbsp. water sweetened with saccharine. Tea.

Protein 53 grams, Fat 100 grams, Carbohydrate 15 grams, Calories 1208.

Patient discharged with advice as to diet.

FOOD VALUES.

An estimate of the quantity of bulk of food may be of assistance or interest. There is so much variation in the size of tablespoons or what may be termed either rounding or heaping tablespoons that it must be remembered that we can only estimate. Patients who are instructed how to feed themselves on leaving the hospital are cautioned carefully to take about the quantity of an article of food they have been served while in the hospital when the diet is weighed. Any written advice is always given in quantities known to be under the carbohydrate or protein tolerance of the patient. However, if they will boil the vegetables and change the water at least twice, so much carbohydrate is removed that it is quite possible for them to obtain a comfortable bulk and still take in very small quantities of carbohydrate.

100-Gram Portions.

Asparagus--8 or 9 stalks 4 inches long. Beans (string) (cut in small pieces) 3 heaping tablespoons. Bacon--4 slices 6 inches long, 2 inches wide.[7] Cabbage (cooked)--3 heaping tablespoons. Cauliflower--3 rounding tablespoons. Celery--6 pieces 4-1/2 inches long, medium thickness. Cheese--a piece 4 inches by 1-1/2 inch by 1 inch. Cucumbers--12 slices 1/8 inch thick, 1/2 inch in diameter. Greens (spinach, kale, etc.)--2 heaping tablespoons. Lettuce--10 to 12 medium-sized leaves. Onions--2 onions, size of an egg. Olives--25 small olives. Peas--3 rounding tablespoons. Potatoes (baked)--1 small potato, size of egg. Potatoes (mashed)--2 rounding tablespoons. Sardines--28 sardines--1 small box. Salmon--1/4 can (almost). Tomatoes--2-1/2 heaping tablespoons. Tomatoes--fresh, one medium sized tomato, 2 inches in diameter.

[7] Bacon loses about half of its fat content when cooked.

Other Weights.

1 tablespoon olive oil = 13 grams 1 tablespoon mayonnaise = 21 " 1 thin slice of bread (baker's loaf) = 25 " 1 medium sized orange = 150 " 1 peach = 125 " 1 medium sized apple = 150 " 1/2 small grape fruit = 150 " 1 medium sized lamb chop with bone = 100 " 1 medium sized slice cold tongue = 25 " 1 slice tenderloin steak 1 in. thick = 100 " 1 average helping of fish = 100 " 1 average helping of butter = 10 " 1 average sized egg = 50 " 1 average helping of cooked green vegetables such as spinach, cabbage, cauliflower, asparagus, etc. (2 tablespoons)[8] = 100 " 1 average helping boiled cereal = 100 " 1 potato, size of large egg = 100 "

[8] It is not true that all the vegetables weigh the same, but for the sake of simplicity in most of the diets it has been reckoned that two heaping tablespoons of any one of the "5%" vegetables weighs 100 gms.

The following food values are taken from Locke's Abstract of Atwater and Bryant's Bulletin No. 28, 1906, United States Department of Agriculture.

Fractions of per cents. have been left off in order to make the use of the table more simple, and the values given will be found quite accurate enough for clinical purposes.

Food Stuffs. Quantity. Protein. Fat. Carbohydrate. Total Raw. Grams. Grams. Grams. Calories.

MEAT.

Beef 100 gms. 22 28 350 Chicken " " 32 4 168 Bacon (raw) " " 10 64 636

FISH.

Fish (average) " " 20 7 147 Oysters " " 6 1 3 46

EGGS.

Eggs " " 13 12 165 Eggs 1 egg 7 6 84

DAIRY PRODUCTS.

Butter 100 gms. 1 85 795 Cheese (American) " " 28 35 2 448 Cheese (Neufch鈚 el) " " 19 27 2 337 Milk (whole) " " 3 4 5 70 Milk (whole) 1 qt. 30 36 45 642 Milk (skim) 100 gms. 3 0.3 5 35 Milk (skim) 1 qt. 31 3 46 343 Cream (gravity) 100 gms. 3 16 5 181 Cream (gravity) 1 pt. 12 73 23 822

CEREAL PRODUCTS.

Oatmeal (cooked) 100 gms. 3 0.5 12 66 Rice (cooked) " " 3 0.1 24 112 Macaroni (cooked) " " 3 0.1 24 112 Bread " " 9 1 53 264 Soda crackers " " 10 9 73 424 Cake (average) " " 6 9 63 367

VEGETABLES.

Asparagus (canned) 100 gms. 2 1 3 30 Beans (dried) " " 22 2 59 350 Beans (string) fresh cooked " " 1 1.0 2 22 Beets (cooked) " " 2 0.1 7 37 Cabbage (raw) " " 2 0.3 6 35 Carrots (raw) " " 1 0.4 9 45 Cauliflower (raw) " " 2 0.5 5 33 Celery (raw) " " 1 0.1 3 17 Corn (green) " " 3 1 20 103 Cucumbers (raw) " " 0.8 0.2 3 17 Lettuce (raw) " " 1 0.3 3 19 Mushrooms (raw) " " 3 0.4 7 45 Onions (raw) " " 1 0.3 10 48 Peas (dried) " " 24 1 62 362 Peas (green, raw) " " 7 0.5 16

99 Potatoes (white) " " 2 0.1 18 83 Potatoes (sweet) " " 2 0.7 27 125 Spinach " " 2 0.3 3 23 Squash " " 1 0.5 9 46 Tomatoes " " 0.9 0.4 4 24 Turnips " " 1 0.2 8 39

The values for all the vegetables are calculated from the raw vegetables.

FRUITS.

Apples (edible portion) 100 gms. 0.4 0.5 14 64 Bananas (edible portion) " " 1 0.6 22 100 Blackberries " " 1 1 11 59 Cherries " " 0.1 1 15 71 Cranberries 100 gms. 0.4 0.6 10 48 Currants " " 1 13 57 Figs (dried) " " 4 0.3 74 323 Grapes " " 1 1 14 71 Huckleberries " " 0.6 0.6 16 74 Lemon juice " " 10 41 Muskmelons (edible portions) " " 0.6 9 39 Oranges (edible portion) " " 0.8 0.2 11 50 Peaches (edible portion) " " 0.7 0.1 9 41 Pears (edible portion) " " 0.6 0.5 14 65 Prunes (dried) " " 2 73 308 Raisins (dried) " " 2 3 76 348 Pineapples " " 0.4 0.3 10 45 Plums (edible portion) " " 1 20 86 Raspberries " " 1 12 53 Strawberries " " 1 0.6 7 38 Watermelons " " 0.4 0.2 7 32

NUTS.

Almonds. 100 gms. 21 54 17 658 Chestnuts " " 6 5 42 243 Peanuts (edible portion) " " 25 38 24 554 Walnuts " " 18 64 13 722

MISCELLANEOUS.

Chocolate 100 gms. 13 48 30 623 Whiskey 50 c.c. 43% alcohol 152 Lager beer 250 c.c. 4.5% alcohol 130

ADDITIONAL DATA.

Protein. Fat. Carbohydrate. Calories.

Bacon (raw) 4 slices, 6 in. long 2 in. wide 10 64 636 Bacon (cooked) 4 slices, 6 in. long, 2 in. wide 10 32 338 to 46 to 468 Beef (roast), 1 slice, 4-1/2 x 1-1/2 x 1/8 in. 6 7 89 Egg, 1 medium size, 50 gms. 7 6 84 Oysters, 6 large 6 1 3 46 Butter, 1-1/4 in. cube (25 gms.) 21 195 Cheese (Neufch 鉳 el) 1 cheese 2-1/4 x 1-1/2 x 1-1/4 in. 16 23 1 284 Cream (gravity--"16%"), 1 glass, 7 oz. 5 32 10 359 Milk (whole), 1 glass, 7 oz. 6 8 9 136 Bread, 1 slice, 3 x 3-1/2 x 1/2 in. (30 gms.) 3 0.5 16 81 Uneeda Biscuit (1) 1 0.5 4 20 Rice (boiled), 1 tablespoon, (50 gms.) 1+ 12 56 Oatmeal (boiled), 1 tablespoon, (50 gms.) 1+ + 6 33 Potato (size of large egg), 100 gms. 2 + 18 83 "5%" vegetables (uncooked) 1 tablespoon 2.5 10 "5%" vegetables (boiled once) 1 tablespoon 1.7 7 "5%" vegetables (boiled thrice) 1 tablespoon 1 4 Grape fruit as purchased (1 small) 300 gms. 2 30 131 Orange as purchased (1 medium) 150 gms. 1 13 57 English walnuts (6 whole meats) 20 gms. 4 12 3 140 Almonds (10 small) 10 gms. 2 5 2 63 Peanuts (as purchased) 15 nuts 6 9 6 33

All of these values are approximate. The following vegetables may be considered as falling into the "5%" group: Lettuce, string beans, spinach, cabbage, Brussels sprouts, egg plant, cauliflower, tomatoes, asparagus, cucumbers, beet greens, chard, celery, Sauerkraut, ripe olives, kale, rhubarb, dandelions, endive, watercress, pumpkin, sorrel, and radishes. As these various vegetables contain from 3 to 7% carbohydrate, it will be seen that the value of 2-1/2 grams carbohydrate for 1 tablespoonful of these vegetables raw, and 1 gram for the same amount thrice boiled, is not accurate, but it is near enough for practical purposes.

###